THE INFLAMMATION SOLUTION.

Harness the Healing Power of an Anti-Inflammatory Lifestyle.

Lois T. Jeffers

Table of Contents

INTRODUCTION

Inflammation, commonly portrayed as the body's natural response to damage or infection, is a complicated biological process that is essential for overall health and well-being. At its core, inflammation is the body's defensive mechanism, organizing a complex network of cellular and molecular interactions to protect against damaging stimuli and promote tissue healing. When inflammation becomes chronic or dysregulated, it can lead to the development of a variety of diseases, including cardiovascular disease, autoimmune problems, and even cancer. Understanding the fundamental causes of inflammation is critical for determining its function in health and illness. This introduction seeks to clarify the idea of inflammation by investigating its physiological origin, triggers, and consequences for human health.

The Role of Diet in Inflammation

Diet plays a critical function in controlling inflammation in the body. According to research, various foods can either promote or reduce inflammation, emphasizing the importance of dietary choices in overall health. A diet high in processed foods, refined sugars, and unhealthy fats has been linked to elevated inflammation, which contributes to the onset and progression of chronic diseases like obesity, type 2 diabetes, and cardiovascular disease.

In contrast, integrating anti-inflammatory items into one's diet can help reduce inflammation and promote optimal health. These include nutrient-dense fruits and vegetables like berries, leafy greens, and cruciferous vegetables, which are high in antioxidants and phytonutrients that have been shown to reduce inflammation. Furthermore, foods high in omega-3 fatty acids, such as fatty fish, flaxseeds, and walnuts, have powerful anti-inflammatory qualities and can help regulate the body's inflammatory response.

Furthermore, dietary patterns such as the Mediterranean diet, which emphasizes plant-based foods, healthy fats, and lean proteins, have been demonstrated to reduce inflammation indicators and lessen the risk of chronic diseases. Individuals who follow a balanced and nutritious diet can use nutrition to manage inflammation, promote healing, and protect themselves from the negative consequences of chronic inflammation on health.

Benefits of an Anti-Inflammatory Diet

Adopting an anti-inflammatory diet provides numerous benefits that go beyond just lowering inflammation. Here are several major advantages:

<u>Lowered Risk of Chronic Disease</u>: An anti-inflammatory diet, by reducing inflammation, can reduce the risk of chronic illnesses like heart disease, diabetes, and some malignancies. It contributes to maintaining optimal levels of inflammation, which promotes general health and longevity.

<u>Weight management:</u> An anti-inflammatory diet often focuses on full, nutrient-dense meals while restricting processed and high-calorie options. This strategy promotes good weight management and can help reduce obesity-related inflammation.

<u>Improved Gut Health:</u> Many anti-inflammatory foods, such as fruits, vegetables, and fermented foods, help to maintain a healthy gut microbiome. A well-balanced gut microbiota is linked to decreased inflammation and enhanced digestive function.

<u>Increased Immune Function:</u> Chronic inflammation can weaken the immune system, leaving people more vulnerable to infections and disorders. An anti-inflammatory diet boosts immune function and the body's ability to combat pathogens by consuming foods high in vitamins, minerals, and antioxidants.

<u>Improved joint health:</u> Inflammatory joint disorders, such as arthritis, can have a substantial impact on mobility and quality of life. An anti-inflammatory diet, particularly one high in omega-3 fatty acids and antioxidants, may help relieve joint pain and stiffness, hence improving total joint function.

<u>Mental Wellbeing:</u> Recent study reveals a relationship between inflammation and mental health issues like sadness and anxiety. An anti-inflammatory diet may improve mood and cognitive performance by lowering systemic inflammation, hence enhancing mental health.

CHAPTER 1: UNDERSTANDING INFLAMMATION

Understanding how inflammation works is critical on the path to well-being. This chapter goes deeply into the complexity of inflammation, examining its physiological mechanisms, triggers, and health consequences. By describing the fundamental principles of inflammation, readers will acquire vital insights into how this critical biological process influences our bodies' reactions to injury, infection, and illness. This chapter seeks to provide readers with knowledge that can be used to inform preventative tactics, therapeutic interventions, and lifestyle choices that promote optimal health and well-being.

Types of Inflammation

Inflammation can take many different forms, each with its own set of traits and underlying causes. Understanding the many forms of inflammation is critical for properly identifying and treating inflammatory disorders. Here are some of the main types:

Acute inflammation

Acute inflammation is the body's immediate and localized response to an injury, infection, or tissue damage. It is a finely controlled process involving a series of molecular and cellular activities targeted at restoring tissue homeostasis and encouraging healing. Understanding the complex mechanisms that drive acute inflammation provides important insights into its involvement in health and disease. Here are some crucial elements to consider:

- Initiation and Triggers: The innate immune system recognizes damaging stimuli such as infections, physical trauma, or chemical irritants, which initiates acute inflammation. This identification causes the production of signaling molecules, like as cytokines and chemokines that orchestrate the inflammatory response.
- Vascular Changes: One of the distinguishing characteristics of acute inflammation is fast dilatation of blood vessels (vasodilation) and enhanced vascular permeability. These alterations allow immune cells like neutrophils and macrophages to move from the bloodstream to the site of damage or infection, where they can help eliminate pathogens and debris.
- Cellular Events: Once at the site of inflammation, immune cells engage in a series of dynamic interactions with the surrounding tissue. Neutrophils are among the first responders, vigorously phagocytozing infections and secreting antimicrobial compounds. Macrophages perform a crucial function in absorbing cellular debris and coordinating the resolution of inflammation.

> **Inflammatory Mediators**: Acute inflammation causes the release of a variety of inflammatory mediators such as prostaglandins, leukotrienes, and histamine. These chemicals contribute to inflammation's hallmark symptoms, such as redness, heat, swelling, and pain, as well as helping to coordinate immune cell recruitment and activation.

> **Resolution and Tissue Repair**: Acute inflammation is a self-limiting process that is carefully controlled to avoid excessive tissue damage. When the inciting stimulus is eliminated or neutralized, anti-inflammatory signals promote inflammation resolution and the start of tissue repair processes such as angiogenesis, collagen deposition, and wound healing.

Clinical Implications: While acute inflammation is an important component of the body's defense mechanisms, deregulation or persistence of acute inflammation can lead to the development of a variety of disorders. Excessive acute inflammation is linked to illnesses including sepsis, acute respiratory distress syndrome (ARDS), and ischemia-reperfusion damage.

Granulomatous Inflammation.

Granulomatous inflammation is a type of chronic inflammation distinguished by the formation of granulomas, which are organized groupings of immune cells called macrophages.

Understanding the complexities of granulomatous inflammation reveals important information about its origins, clinical presentations, and consequences for health and illness. Here are some crucial elements to consider:

- <u>Granuloma Formation</u>: Granulomas are organized groups of immune cells, primarily macrophages that are surrounded by a rim of lymphocytes. These organized structures emerge in response to persistent or incompletely destroyed infections, foreign chemicals, or changed self-antigens that the immune system is unable to eliminate. Granulomas act as a protective mechanism by containing and neutralizing these stimuli, stopping their spread, and reducing tissue damage.

- <u>Cellular Components</u>: Macrophages play an important role in the development and maintenance of granulomatous inflammation. When exposed to the inciting stimulus, macrophages activate and aggregate, forming the core of the granuloma. Other immune cells, such as lymphocytes, multinucleated giant cells, and fibroblasts, may also contribute to the creation and function of granulomas.

- <u>Underlying Causes</u>: Granulomatous inflammation can result from a variety of viral and non-infectious sources.

- Infectious causes include mycobacterial diseases (e.g., tuberculosis, leprosy), fungal infections (e.g., histoplasmosis, cryptococcosis), and parasite infections. Non-infectious causes include autoimmune illnesses

> (sarcoidosis, granulomatosis with polyangiitis), foreign body reactions, and granulomatous medication reactions.

> ‣ <u>Etiology:</u> The etiology of granulomatous inflammation is complex, involving immune responses, cytokine signaling, and tissue remodeling. Persistent antigen stimulation recruits and activates macrophages, which then produce pro-inflammatory cytokines and chemokines, thus sustaining the inflammatory response. Granulomas can fibrosis and calcify over time, resulting in tissue damage and organ failure.

Clinical Manifestations: The clinical manifestations of granulomatous inflammation differ based on the underlying etiology and the organs involved. Common symptoms include fever, weight loss, exhaustion, respiratory symptoms (such as coughing and dyspnea), skin lesions, and organ malfunction. Clinical evaluation, imaging examinations (e.g., chest X-ray, CT scan), laboratory testing, and histological analysis of tissue biopsies are frequently used in the diagnosis process.

Treatment and Management: The management of granulomatous inflammation is determined by the underlying etiology and the degree of symptoms. Antimicrobial therapy may be required in infectious cases to eliminate the organism and alleviate inflammation.

Corticosteroids and disease-modifying anti-rheumatic medications (DMARDs) are two immunosuppressive medicines that are often used to manage inflammation in autoimmune illnesses.

In some circumstances, surgical intervention may be necessary to remove granulomatous lesions or relieve organ compression.

Continuing research efforts to elucidate the immunological basis of granuloma formation show promise for the development of specific therapy techniques to control the inflammatory response and improve outcomes for affected people.

Allergic Inflammation

Allergic inflammation is a complicated immunological response defined by hypersensitivity to innocuous chemicals known as allergens. Understanding the complex mechanisms that underpin allergic inflammation provides insights into the development, clinical symptoms, and treatment of allergic disorders. Here are some crucial elements to consider:

> Immunological Sensitization: Allergic inflammation usually begins with immunological sensitization, a process in which the immune system becomes reactive to certain allergens. During sensitization, antigen-presenting cells, such as dendritic cells, detect allergens and present them to T cells, activating allergen-specific T-helper 2 (Th2) cells.
> Th2 cells release cytokines such as interleukin-4 (IL-4), interleukin-5 (IL-5), and interleukin-13 (IL-13), which stimulate B cells to create allergen-specific IgE antibodies.

- Instant Hypersensitivity Reaction: When exposed to the allergen again, IgE antibodies bind to mast cells and basophils, causing an instant hypersensitivity reaction. Cross-linking of IgE receptors on these cells causes the production of inflammatory mediators such as histamine, leukotrienes, and prostaglandins, which cause vasodilation, increased vascular permeability, smooth muscle contraction, and inflammatory cell recruitment. This acute phase reaction causes quick onset of symptoms such as itching, hives, edema, and bronchoconstriction.

- Late-Phase Reaction: In addition to the acute hypersensitive reaction, allergic inflammation can be followed by a late-phase reaction, which involves the recruitment of eosinophils, neutrophils, and other inflammatory cells to the site of allergen exposure. This delayed inflammatory response is responsible for the persistence of symptoms and tissue damage, especially in chronic allergic disorders like asthma, allergic rhinitis, and atopic dermatitis.

- Airway Inflammation in Asthma: Allergic inflammation is a key factor in the development of asthma, a chronic respiratory illness marked by airway inflammation, bronchial hyper responsiveness, and reversible airflow restriction. Inhaled allergens activate the cells and cause the release of pro-inflammatory cytokines, resulting in airway eosinophilia, mucus hypersecretion, and smooth muscle contraction.

Asthma care relies heavily on anti-inflammatory drugs like inhaled corticosteroids and leukotriene modifiers to combat allergic inflammation.

- ▹ <u>Atopic March and Allergic Comorbidities:</u> Allergic inflammation is frequently connected with a condition known as the atopic march, in which individuals with allergic disorders such as eczema (atopic dermatitis) in infancy may acquire allergic rhinitis and asthma later in childhood. Allergic inflammation can also lead to the development of additional allergic comorbidities such as food allergies, allergic conjunctivitis, and allergic sinusitis.

- ▹ <u>Management Strategies:</u> The treatment of allergic inflammation includes allergen avoidance, medication, and immunomodulatory treatments. Allergen avoidance tactics include environmental alterations, allergen immunotherapy (allergy shots), and targeted avoidance measures. Antihistamines, corticosteroids, leukotriene receptor antagonists, mast cell stabilizers, and biological medicines that target specific inflammatory pathways are all part of pharmacotherapy.

Chronic Inflammation

Chronic inflammation is a prolonged and dysregulated immune response that can last weeks, months, or even years. Unlike acute inflammation, which is a temporary protective reaction, chronic inflammation can cause tissue damage and contribute to the development of numerous chronic diseases. Exploring the complexity of chronic inflammation reveals its multidimensional character and the consequences for health and disease. Here are some crucial aspects to explore further:

- ▹ <u>Underlying Mechanisms:</u> Chronic inflammation results from a complex interaction of genetic, environmental, and behavioral variables. Prolonged exposure to inflammatory stimuli, such as infections, environmental pollutants, dietary variables, and metabolic abnormalities, can maintain and exacerbate the inflammatory response. Dysregulation of immune cells, cytokines, and signaling pathways all contribute to the chronic inflammatory state.

- ▹ <u>Systemic Effects:</u> Unlike acute inflammation, which is typically localized, chronic inflammation can present systemically, impacting various organs and tissues across the body. Systemic inflammation is defined by heightened levels of circulating inflammatory markers such as C-reactive protein (CRP), interleukin-6 (IL-6), and tumor necrosis factor-alpha (TNF-alpha), which are linked to an increased risk of chronic illnesses.

- ▹ <u>Contributing Factors:</u> Chronic inflammation is linked to the development of many chronic diseases, including cardiovascular disease, type 2 diabetes, obesity, autoimmune disorders, neurodegenerative diseases, and some malignancies. Inflammatory processes play an important role in the development and progression of many diseases, including tissue damage, insulin resistance, abnormal immunological responses, and tumor growth.

- <u>Immunological Imbalance:</u> Chronic inflammation is defined by a persistent imbalance of pro-inflammatory and anti-inflammatory pathways. While pro-inflammatory cytokines and immune cells initiate the inflammatory response, anti-inflammatory mediators like interleukin-10 (IL-10) and transforming growth factor-beta (TGF-beta) work to reduce inflammation and restore tissue homeostasis. Dysregulation of this equilibrium can exacerbate chronic inflammation and contribute to disease etiology.

- <u>Clinical Manifestations:</u> The clinical manifestations of chronic inflammation differ based on the underlying disease and the tissues involved. Fatigue, joint discomfort, muscular stiffness, cognitive impairment, gastrointestinal abnormalities, and skin manifestations are all potential symptoms. Chronic inflammatory disorders frequently follow a relapsing-remitting pattern, with episodes of exacerbation and remission.

- <u>Therapeutic Strategies:</u> Combating chronic inflammation is a viable therapeutic technique for controlling chronic diseases and improving health outcomes. Lifestyle changes, such as eating an anti-inflammatory diet, exercising regularly, managing stress, and quitting smoking, can all help reduce chronic inflammation. Pharmacological therapies, such as anti-inflammatory medications and biologic medicines that target specific inflammatory pathways, are also used to reduce inflammation and slow disease development.

Causes of Chronic Inflammation

Chronic inflammation can be caused by a wide range of circumstances, including lifestyle choices and underlying medical disorders. The following are some common causes of chronic inflammation:

1. Poor Diet.

A poor diet, which includes processed foods, high quantities of refined carbohydrates, bad fats, and chemicals, contributes significantly to chronic inflammation. Understanding the complex link between nutrition and inflammation sheds light on the mechanisms by which dietary variables affect immune function, metabolic health, and disease risk. Here are some crucial elements to consider:

<u>Pro-inflammatory Foods:</u> Processed foods, such as sugary snacks, refined grains, fried foods, and processed meats, frequently contain pro-inflammatory substances such as trans-fats, refined carbohydrates, and additives. These foods may cause inflammation by increasing oxidative stress, insulin resistance, and dyslipidemia.

<u>Gut Microbiota Dysbiosis:</u> Poor eating habits can upset the balance of good and dangerous bacteria in the gut, resulting in dysbiosis and intestinal inflammation. Diets low in fiber-rich fruits, vegetables, and whole grains deplete the gut microbiota of vital nutrients, whereas high-fat and high-sugar diets encourage the proliferation of pro-inflammatory bacteria.

<u>Advanced Glycation End Products (AGEs)</u>: Cooking at high temperatures, such as grilling, frying, and broiling, can result in advanced glycation end products (AGEs), which are pro-inflammatory substances created when sugars combine with proteins or fats. AGEs accumulate in tissues, causing chronic inflammation, oxidative stress, and tissue damage.

<u>Omega-6 to Omega-3 Imbalance:</u> The Western diet is heavy in omega-6 fatty acids found in vegetable oils (e.g., corn oil, soybean oil), which can cause inflammation if ingested in excess. In contrast, omega-3 fatty acids found in fatty fish, flaxseeds, and walnuts are anti-inflammatory. An imbalance of omega-6 and omega-3 fatty acids might worsen chronic inflammation.

<u>Adipose Tissue Inflammation:</u> Excess calorie consumption, particularly from refined carbs and harmful fats, can cause adipose tissue growth and adipocyte malfunction. Adipocytes that are enlarged release pro-inflammatory adipokines like tumor necrosis factor-alpha (TNF-alpha) and interleukin-6 (IL-6), which contribute to systemic inflammation and metabolic dysfunction.

<u>Insulin Resistance</u>: Diets high in refined sugars and carbs can lead to insulin resistance, a condition in which cells become less sensitive to insulin's actions. Insulin resistance is linked to chronic inflammation because high levels of circulating glucose and insulin can activate inflammatory pathways, contributing to the development of metabolic syndrome and type 2 diabetes.

<u>Antioxidant Deficiency</u>: A low intake of antioxidant-rich foods such as fruits, vegetables, nuts, and seeds might decrease the body's ability to neutralize reactive oxygen species (ROS) and combat oxidative stress. Chronic oxidative stress can exacerbate inflammation and contribute to the progression of inflammatory disorders.

2. Obesity

Obesity is a complex metabolic condition defined by excessive adipose tissue buildup that is intimately associated with chronic inflammation. Understanding the complex link between obesity and inflammation sheds light on the mechanisms that underpin obesity-related problems and opens up possibilities for targeted therapies. Here are some crucial elements to consider:

> <u>Adipose Tissue Inflammation</u>: Adipose tissue is not only an inactive energy storage depot, but also an active endocrine organ that secretes a variety of adipokines, cytokines, and inflammatory mediators.
> Obesity causes adipocyte malfunction and increased release of pro-inflammatory adipokines such as tumor necrosis factor-alpha (TNF-alpha), interleukin-6 (IL-6), and leptin. Chronic low-grade inflammation in adipose tissue adds to overall inflammation and metabolic dysfunction.

‣ <u>Macrophage Infiltration</u>: Obesity causes a shift in the adipose tissue milieu, marked by increased infiltration of pro-inflammatory immune cells, notably macrophages. These adipose tissue macrophages (ATMs) cause adipose tissue inflammation by secreting pro-inflammatory cytokines and chemokines, which promote insulin resistance and decrease adipocyte function.

‣ <u>Insulin Resistance</u>: Chronic inflammation in obesity disrupts insulin signaling pathways, resulting in insulin resistance, a defining trait of obesity-related metabolic problems such as type 2 diabetes. Pro-inflammatory cytokines, particularly TNF-alpha and IL-6, can activate serine kinases that phosphorylate insulin receptor substrates, reducing insulin receptor signaling and glucose absorption in target organs.

‣ <u>Oxidative Stress</u>: Obesity is linked to increased oxidative stress, which is defined by an imbalance between reactive oxygen species (ROS) production and antioxidant defenses. Adipose tissue inflammation and dysregulated lipid metabolism in obesity contribute to ROS production, resulting in oxidative damage to lipids, proteins, and DNA.

Chronic oxidative stress worsens inflammation and increases the risk of obesity-related comorbidities like cardiovascular disease and nonalcoholic fatty liver disease (NAFLD).

‣ <u>Gut Microbiota Dysbiosis</u>: Obesity alters the composition and function of the gut microbiota, a complex ecosystem of bacteria that live in the gastrointestinal tract.

Dysbiosis is characterized by a decrease in beneficial bacteria and an increase in harmful species, which can lead to inflammation and metabolic failure. Gut-derived microbial compounds, such as lipopolysaccharides (LPS), can enter the bloodstream and cause systemic inflammation and metabolic endotoxemia in obesity.

▸ <u>Systemic Inflammation</u>: Chronic low-grade inflammation in obesity affects more than just adipose tissue; it also affects the liver, skeletal muscle, pancreas, and vascular endothelium. Systemic inflammation has a role in the development of obesity-related comorbidities such as cardiovascular disease, stroke, hypertension, dyslipidemia, and some malignancies.

3. Smoking

Cigarette smoking is a well-known risk factor for chronic inflammation and has been linked to a wide range of inflammatory disorders. Understanding the processes by which smoking causes inflammation sheds light on the etiology of smoking-related illnesses and helps to influence preventative and intervention measures. Here are some crucial elements to consider:

▸ <u>Toxin inhalation:</u> Cigarette smoke includes about 7,000 compounds, many of which are hazardous and carcinogenic. Inhaling these substances, which include nicotine, tar, carbon monoxide, formaldehyde, and heavy metals, causes inflammation in the respiratory tract and systemic circulation. The intake of smoke particles and chemicals directly destroys lung tissue, causing inflammation and oxidative stress.

- Airway Inflammation: Smoking is a key risk factor for respiratory disorders such as chronic obstructive pulmonary disease (COPD), emphysema, and bronchitis, which are characterized by chronic inflammation and restricted airflow. Cigarette smoke irritates and inflames the airway epithelium, causing excessive mucus production, airway remodeling, and neutrophilic inflammation. Chronic airway inflammation causes respiratory symptoms such as coughing, sputum production, wheezing, and dyspnea.
- Alveolar Damage: Smoking-induced inflammation harms alveolar epithelial cells and hinders alveolar repair mechanisms, resulting in alveolar breakdown and airspace enlargement typical of emphysema. Inflammatory mediators such as matrix metalloproteinases (MMPs), interleukins, and tumor necrosis factor-alpha (TNF-alpha) induce tissue remodeling, fibrosis, and apoptosis in the lung parenchyma.
- Systemic Inflammation: Smoking-induced inflammation spreads beyond the respiratory tract and affects systemic circulation, contributing to the development of cardiovascular disease, atherosclerosis, and metabolic syndrome. Cigarette smoke components cause endothelial dysfunction, oxidative stress, and inflammation in vascular endothelial cells, which promotes the production of atherosclerotic plaques and thrombus.

Systemic inflammation also exacerbates insulin resistance and dyslipidemia, which raises the risk of cardiovascular disease and type 2 diabetes.

⮚ Immunological Dysregulation: Smoking impairs immunological function and alters inflammatory pathways, weakening host defenses and increasing vulnerability to infections and autoimmune disorders. Cigarette smoke inhibits immune cell activity, phagocytosis, and cytokine synthesis, resulting in decreased pathogen clearance and dysregulated immunological responses.

⮚ Cancer-Related Inflammation: Smoking is the greatest cause of preventable cancer worldwide, and it is linked to an increased risk of lung cancer, as well as cancers of the mouth, throat, esophagus, pancreas, bladder, and uterus. Cigarette smoke causes chronic inflammation, which increases oncogenic processes such as DNA damage, cell proliferation, angiogenesis, and metastasis, hence contributing to tumor start and progression.

4. Physical Inactivity

Physical inactivity, defined as sedentary behavior and a lack of regular exercise, contributes significantly to chronic inflammation and is linked to an increased risk of inflammatory illnesses. Understanding the processes by which physical inactivity causes inflammation sheds light on the etiology of sedentary-related illnesses and helps to inform preventative and intervention measures. Here are some crucial elements to consider:

- Adipose Tissue Dysfunction: Physical inactivity is linked to increased adiposity and changes in adipose tissue metabolism, resulting in adipocyte dysfunction and the release of pro-inflammatory adipokines like tumor necrosis factor-alpha (TNF-alpha), interleukin-6 (IL-6), and leptin. Excess adipose tissue, particularly visceral fat, causes chronic low-grade inflammation and systemic metabolic dysregulation.
- Insulin Resistance: Sedentary behavior and a lack of exercise contribute to insulin resistance, which is defined by decreased insulin signaling and glucose uptake in target tissues. Physical inactivity-induced insulin resistance is linked to higher levels of circulating glucose and insulin, which can activate inflammatory pathways and increase chronic inflammation.
- Systemic Inflammation: Physical inactivity is linked to higher levels of circulating inflammatory markers such as CRP, IL-6, and TNF-alpha.
  Sedentary behavior stimulates immune cell activation and cytokine production, resulting in persistent low-grade inflammation and endothelial damage. Systemic inflammation promotes the development of inflammatory disorders such as cardiovascular disease, type 2 diabetes, and metabolic syndrome.
- Oxidative Stress: Physical inactivity causes oxidative stress, which is defined by an imbalance between reactive oxygen species (ROS) production and antioxidant

defenses. Sedentary behavior alters mitochondrial function, reduces antioxidant enzyme activity, and enhances ROS production, which causes oxidative damage to lipids, proteins, and DNA. Chronic oxidative stress worsens inflammation and contributes to the development of sedentary-related illnesses.

> Immunological Dysregulation: Regular exercise is crucial for modifying immunological function and encouraging anti-inflammatory responses. Physical inactivity weakens immune surveillance mechanisms and affects immune cell function, making you more susceptible to infections and autoimmune illnesses. Sedentary behavior induces immunological dysregulation, which contributes to chronic inflammation and inflammatory consequences.

> Gut Microbiota Dysbiosis: Physical inactivity alters the makeup and diversity of the gut microbiota, a complex ecosystem of microorganisms that live in the gastrointestinal tract.

> Sedentary behavior causes dysbiosis, which is defined by a decrease in beneficial bacteria and an increase in harmful species, resulting in inflammation and metabolic failure. Lipopolysaccharides (LPS), a type of microbial product found in the gut, can enter the bloodstream and cause inflammation and metabolic endotoxemia.

5. Chronic Stress.

Chronic stress, defined as extended exposure to psychological or environmental stressors, is a major contributor to chronic inflammation and has been linked to an increased risk of inflammatory illnesses. Understanding the processes by which chronic stress causes inflammation sheds light on the etiology of stress-related diseases and helps to influence preventative and therapeutic measures. Here are some crucial elements to consider:

- Hypothalamic-Pituitary-Adrenal (HPA) Axis Dysregulation: Chronic stress activates the hypothalamic-pituitary-adrenal (HPA) axis, causing stress hormones including cortisol and catecholamines to be released. Prolonged activation of the HPA axis disrupts cortisol secretion patterns, resulting in increased cortisol levels and poor negative feedback inhibition. Cortisol signaling dysregulation relates to immunological dysfunction and chronic inflammation.

- Sympathetic Nervous System Activation: Chronic stress stimulates the sympathetic nervous system (SNS), which causes the release of catecholamines like adrenaline and norepinephrine. Sympathetic activation raises heart rate, blood pressure, and peripheral vasoconstriction, priming the body for a "fight or flight" reaction. Prolonged sympathetic activity can lead to cardiovascular disease, immunological dysregulation, and systemic inflammation.

- Glucocorticoid Resistance: Chronic stress-induced dysregulation of the HPA axis can result in glucocorticoid resistance, which is defined as diminished sensitivity of target tissues to cortisol's anti-inflammatory actions. Glucocorticoid resistance causes inadequate regulation of pro-inflammatory cytokines and chemokines, resulting in chronic low-grade inflammation and tissue damage.
- Chronic stress activates immune cells, including monocytes, macrophages, and lymphocytes, resulting in increased production of pro-inflammatory cytokines such as IL-6, TNF-alpha, and IL-1β. Dysregulated cytokine signaling causes chronic inflammation and plays a role in the development of stress-related disorders such as depression, anxiety, and autoimmune diseases.
- Microglial Activation: Chronic stress-induced inflammation in the central nervous system (CNS) results in the activation of microglial cells, the brain's resident immune cells. Activated microglia produce pro-inflammatory cytokines and reactive oxygen species (ROS), resulting in neuro-inflammation, synaptic dysfunction, and neuronal injury. Chronic neuro-inflammation is linked to the development of stress-related mental illnesses and neurodegenerative diseases.
- Allostatic Load: Chronic stress contributes to allostatic load, which is a condition of chronic physiological dysregulation characterized by persistent activation of stress response mechanisms.

Allostatic load refers to the cumulative wear and tear on the body's regulatory systems, which include the neuroendocrine, immunological, and cardiovascular systems, caused by chronic stress exposure. Allostatic load causes chronic inflammation, metabolic inefficiency, and increased disease vulnerability.

6. Environmental Toxins

Environmental toxins are a diverse group of pollutants, chemicals, heavy metals, and contaminants found in the air, water, soil, food, and consumer products. Chronic exposure to environmental pollutants contributes significantly to chronic inflammation and increases the risk of inflammatory disorders. Understanding the processes by which environmental toxins cause inflammation sheds light on the etiology of toxin-related illnesses and helps to influence preventative and therapeutic methods. Here are some crucial elements to consider:

> ➤ <u>Air Pollution</u>: Ambient air pollution, which includes particulate matter (PM), nitrogen dioxide (NO2), sulfur dioxide (SO2), ozone (O3), and volatile organic compounds (VOCs), is a significant environmental toxin linked to systemic inflammation and respiratory disorders. Inhaling air pollutants causes oxidative stress, pulmonary inflammation, and endothelial dysfunction, which leads to respiratory symptoms, worsening of asthma, and an increased risk of cardiovascular events.

- <u>Heavy Metals</u>: Heavy metals like lead, mercury, arsenic, cadmium, and chromium are common environmental contaminants with proven inflammatory effects. Chronic exposure to heavy metals, primarily via contaminated water, soil, and food, boosts oxidative stress, impairs cellular function, and causes inflammation in many organs. Heavy metal-induced inflammation is linked to the development of neurological illnesses, cardiovascular problems, renal dysfunction, and malignancy.

- <u>Pesticides and Herbicides</u>: Pesticides and herbicides, which are widely employed in agriculture and pest control, are highly toxic environmental agents linked to systemic inflammation and immunological dysregulation. Pesticides such as organophosphates, pyrethroids, and glyphosate affect endocrine function, weaken immunological responses, and cause chronic inflammation. Pesticide exposure has been related to an increased risk of neurological problems, autoimmune diseases, and certain malignancies.

- <u>Persistent Organic Pollutants (POPs)</u>: Persistent organic pollutants, such as polychlorinated biphenyls (PCBs), dioxins, and poly-brominated diphenyl ethers (PBDEs), are very stable and bio-accumulative environmental toxins that have extended half-lives in the environment and human body. Chronic exposure to POPs from polluted food, water, and consumer products affects endocrine function, changes immunological responses, and increases chronic inflammation.

POPs are linked to an increased risk of metabolic problems, reproductive abnormalities, and cardiovascular illnesses.

- ⯈ <u>Endocrine Disrupting Chemicals (EDCs):</u> Chemicals that disrupt endocrine function include bisphenol A (BPA), phthalates, parabens, and perfluoroalkyl substances (PFAS). Chronic exposure to EDCs, primarily from plastics, personal care products, and food packaging, leads to systemic inflammation, metabolic dysfunction, and reproductive abnormalities. EDCs are linked to an increased risk of obesity, diabetes, infertility, and hormone-related malignancies.

- ⯈ <u>Indoor Environmental Toxins:</u> Volatile organic compounds (VOCs), formaldehyde, mold, and indoor allergens all contribute to indoor air pollution and poor indoor environmental quality (IEQ). Chronic exposure to indoor pollutants, especially in poorly ventilated areas, can worsen respiratory symptoms, allergic reactions, and inflammatory disorders like asthma and allergic rhinitis.

7. Autoimmune Disorders

Autoimmune disorders are a set of diseases defined by dysregulated immune responses to self-antigens, which cause chronic inflammation and tissue damage. Understanding the processes that drive autoimmune inflammation sheds light on the pathophysiology of autoimmune disorders and informs diagnostic, therapeutic, and management techniques. Here are some crucial elements to consider:

- Loss of Self-Tolerance: Autoimmune illnesses result from a failure in immune tolerance mechanisms, which typically keep the immune system from attacking self-antigens. Genetic predisposition, environmental stressors, and immune checkpoint dysregulation can all contribute to the loss of self-tolerance and the onset of autoimmunity.
- Autoimmune Cascade: The etiology of autoimmune illnesses is a complicated interaction of genetic, environmental, and immunological variables. Autoimmune reactions normally continue through three stages: initiation, amplification, and persistence of the autoimmune cascade. The detection of self-antigens by autoreactive immune cells triggers the activation of T and B cells. Amplification is the proliferation and differentiation of autoreactive lymphocytes, which results in the generation of autoantibodies and pro-inflammatory cytokines. Perpetuation is defined as the ongoing activation of inflammatory pathways and tissue damage that results in the clinical signs of autoimmune disease.
- Inflammatory Mediators: Activated immune cells produce pro-inflammatory cytokines, chemokines, and inflammatory mediators, which define autoimmune inflammation. Cytokines like TNF-alpha, IL-1β, and IL-6 promote inflammation, recruit immune cells to target tissues, and boost immune responses. Inflammatory mediators cause tissue damage, organ dysfunction, and the persistence of autoimmune inflammation.

- Tissue-Specific Autoimmunity: Autoimmune illnesses can attack specific organs or tissues, resulting in either organ-specific or systemic autoimmune diseases. Organ-specific autoimmune illnesses include type 1 diabetes (pancreas), multiple sclerosis (central nervous system), rheumatoid arthritis (joints), and Hashimoto's thyroiditis. Systemic autoimmune illnesses, such as systemic lupus erythematosus (SLE) and systemic sclerosis (scleroderma), include immune responses that affect various organs and tissues throughout the body.

- Immunological Dysregulation: Autoimmune disorders are defined by dysregulated immunological responses, such as abnormal activation of T cells, B cells, and antigen-presenting cells. Dysfunctional regulatory T cells (Tregs) and compromised immunological checkpoints lead to the loss of immune tolerance and the persistence of autoimmune inflammation. Genetic predisposition, environmental triggers (such as infections and toxins), hormonal variables, and epigenetic alterations can all contribute to immune dysregulation.

- Treatment Strategies: The goal of treating autoimmune illnesses is to reduce autoimmune inflammation, alleviate symptoms, and prevent the disease from progressing. Immunosuppressive pharmaceuticals (e.g., corticosteroids, disease-modifying anti-rheumatic drugs, biologic agents), anti-inflammatory drugs, and immunomodulatory therapy are all common treatment options.

Targeted medicines that target specific inflammatory pathways or immune cell targets have transformed the treatment of autoimmune illnesses, increasing results and quality of life for patients.

8. Aging

Aging is a complex biological process defined by a gradual decline in physiological function and an increasing risk of age-related disorders. Chronic inflammation, sometimes known as "inflammaging," is a defining aspect of aging and plays an important role in the pathogenesis of age-related diseases. Understanding the pathways that link aging and inflammation sheds light on the molecular, cellular, and systemic alterations that lead to age-related inflammation, as well as informing healthy aging therapies. Here are some crucial elements to consider:

- Senescence and Immune Dysregulation: Aging is linked to immune system dysregulation, which includes changes in immune cell function, reduced immune surveillance, and poorer immunological responses to infections and antigens. Immunosenescence, or the age-related reduction in immunological function, causes chronic low-grade inflammation and increases vulnerability to infections, autoimmune disorders, and cancer. Senescent cells, which accumulate with age, release pro-inflammatory cytokines, chemokines, and extracellular matrix remodeling enzymes, contributing to chronic inflammation and tissue damage.

▷ Oxidative Stress and Cellular Damage: Aging is associated with increasing oxidative stress, which is caused by an imbalance between reactive oxygen species (ROS) production and antioxidant defenses. ROS-induced oxidative damage to lipids, proteins, and DNA accumulates over time, contributing to cellular and mitochondrial malfunction, as well as genomic instability. Oxidative stress activates inflammatory pathways, causes cellular senescence, and exacerbates age-related inflammation and tissue degradation.

▷ Mitochondrial malfunction: Mitochondrial malfunction is a defining trait of aging and is intimately associated with age-related inflammation. Accumulation of mitochondrial DNA (mtDNA) mutations, decreased mitochondrial biogenesis, and faulty mitochondrial quality control mechanisms all lead to mitochondrial dysfunction and elevated ROS levels. Dysfunctional mitochondria produce mitochondrial-derived damage-associated molecular patterns (DAMPs), which activate innate immune responses and increase inflammation.

▷ Inflammasome Activation: The NLRP3 inflammasome, a multiprotein complex that governs innate immune responses, is linked to age-related inflammation and inflammatory disorders. Activation of the NLRP3 inflammasome in response to cellular stress, DAMPs, and metabolic dysfunction leads to the production of pro-inflammatory cytokines such as interleukin-1 beta (IL-1β) and interleukin-18 (IL-18). Inflammasome-mediated inflammation is linked to age-related illnesses such as neurodegenerative diseases, cardiovascular diseases, and metabolic disorders.

‣ Gut Microbiota Dysbiosis: Aging causes changes in the composition and diversity of the gut microbiota, which is a complex ecosystem of bacteria that live in the gastrointestinal tract. Age-related changes in food, immunological function, and gut physiology all contribute to gut microbiota dysbiosis, which is defined by a decrease in helpful bacteria and an increase in pathogenic species. Dysbiotic gut microbiota increase intestinal permeability, cause systemic inflammation, and contribute to age-related illnesses such as inflammatory bowel disease, cardiovascular disease, and cognitive decline.

‣ Epigenetic Modifications: Aging causes changes in epigenetic regulation, such as DNA methylation, histone modifications, and non-coding RNA expression. Epigenetic changes affect gene expression patterns, cellular differentiation, and aging-related processes such as cellular senescence and inflammation.

Alterations in the epigenome associated with aging contribute to dysregulated immunological responses, increased vulnerability to age-related illnesses, and inflammation.

Symptoms.

Chronic inflammation symptoms vary greatly based on the underlying cause, afflicted organs or tissues, and the individual's health status. While acute inflammation is characterized by conventional indicators such as redness, swelling, heat, and pain, chronic inflammation may be more subtle and persistent. The following are some common signs and manifestations of chronic inflammation.

- Weariness: Chronic inflammation can cause systemic reactions that result in persistent weariness and lethargy. The immune system is active for an extended period, diverting energy resources and adding to fatigue.
- Joint Pain: Chronic inflammation is linked to inflammatory joint conditions such as rheumatoid arthritis, psoriatic arthritis, and ankylosing spondylitis. Chronic inflammation in the joints can cause swelling, stiffness, and discomfort, reducing mobility and quality of life.
- Muscle Aches and Pains: Chronic inflammation can produce generalized muscle aches and pains, commonly known as myalgia. Inflammatory mediators produced during chronic inflammation can cause muscle stiffness, pain, and decreased muscle function.
- Gastrointestinal Symptoms: Chronic inflammation of the gastrointestinal system can cause symptoms such as stomach discomfort, bloating, diarrhea, constipation, and changed bowel patterns.

Inflammatory bowel illnesses (IBD), such as Crohn's disease and ulcerative colitis, are distinguished by chronic inflammation of the intestinal mucosa.

▶ Skin Changes: Chronic inflammation can cause skin symptoms such as redness, swelling, itching, and rash. Eczema, psoriasis, and dermatitis are all conditions characterized by persistent inflammatory responses in the skin, which cause flare-ups and lesions.

▶ Cognitive Impairment: Chronic inflammation has been linked to cognitive decline and neurodegenerative disorders such as Alzheimer's and Parkinson's disease. Inflammatory mediators can pass the blood-brain barrier, causing neuro-inflammation, neuronal damage, and cognitive impairment.

▶ Respiratory Symptoms: Chronic inflammation of the respiratory tract can cause coughing, wheezing, shortness of breath, and chest tightness. Chronic obstructive pulmonary disease (COPD), asthma, and bronchiectasis are all characterized by airway inflammation over time.

▶ Systemic Symptoms: Chronic inflammation can cause fever, lethargy, weight loss, and night sweats. These symptoms are the body's systemic response to ongoing immunological activation and inflammatory signals.

▶ Cardiovascular Symptoms: Chronic inflammation is a key factor in the development of cardiovascular disorders such as atherosclerosis, coronary artery disease, and myocarditis. Symptoms may include angina (chest pain), palpitations, shortness of breath, and exhaustion.

▶ Autoimmune Symptoms: Autoimmune illnesses characterized by persistent inflammation can cause a wide spectrum of symptoms affecting many organs and systems. Common autoimmune symptoms include joint discomfort, fatigue, rash, fever, hair loss, and unexplained weight fluctuations.

CHAPTER 2: ANTI-INFLAMMATORY FOODS

In this chapter, we will look at a variety of nutrient-dense foods that have anti-inflammatory qualities and can help reduce chronic inflammation in the body.

Fruits and Vegetables

Fruits and vegetables are important components of an anti-inflammatory diet because they include a wide range of vitamins, minerals, antioxidants, and phytochemicals. Including a range of colorful fruits and vegetables in your daily meals will help reduce chronic inflammation, boost immunological function, and improve overall health. Take a closer look at the anti-inflammatory qualities of certain fruits and vegetables.

> **Berries:** Berries including strawberries, blueberries, raspberries, and blackberries are high in antioxidants, especially flavonoids, and anthocyanins, which have strong anti-inflammatory properties. These substances serve to neutralize free radicals, minimize oxidative stress, and suppress inflammatory pathways in the body. Berries are also high in fiber, vitamins C and K, and other minerals that promote immunological and cardiovascular health.

> **Leafy Greens**: Dark leafy greens, such as spinach, kale, Swiss chard, and collard greens, are high in vitamins A, C, and K, as well as minerals like calcium and magnesium.

They also contain phytonutrients like carotenoids, flavonoids, and glucosinolates, which are anti-inflammatory and antioxidant. Incorporating leafy greens into salads, soups, smoothies, and stir-fries can help enhance nutrient intake and reduce inflammation.

- **Cruciferous Vegetables:** Cruciferous vegetables, such as broccoli, cauliflower, Brussels sprouts, and cabbage, contain sulfur-containing chemicals called sulforaphane and glucosinolates, which have powerful anti-inflammatory and anti-cancer qualities. These vegetables also contain vitamins, minerals, and fiber, which promote digestive health and immunological function. Regular eating of cruciferous vegetables has been linked to reduced inflammation and a lower risk of chronic diseases.

- **Colorful Vegetables**: Colorful vegetables such as bell peppers, tomatoes, carrots, and sweet potatoes are high in vitamins, minerals, antioxidants, and phytochemicals, which assist in fighting inflammation and oxidative stress. For example, tomatoes contain lycopene, a potent antioxidant with anti-inflammatory qualities, whereas carrots are high in beta-carotene, which is converted to vitamin A in the body and promotes immune function and eye health.

- **Citrus Fruits**: Citrus fruits like oranges, lemons, limes, and grapefruits are high in vitamin C, a powerful antioxidant that reduces inflammation, improves immunological function, and promotes collagen formation. Citrus fruits also include flavonoids and phytochemicals that contribute to their anti-inflammatory benefits.

Consuming citrus fruits and liquids can help decrease inflammatory indicators and improve cardiovascular health.

▷ **Apples:** Apples contain fiber, vitamins, and antioxidants, including quercetin, a flavonoid with anti-inflammatory properties. Quercetin reduces inflammation, stabilizes mast cells, and inhibits the generation of proinflammatory cytokines. Regular consumption of apples and other polyphenol-rich fruits can help regulate immune responses and protect against chronic inflammatory illnesses.

Others: Other anti-inflammatory fruits and vegetables include avocados, cherries, grapes, papayas, pineapple, beets, ginger, and turmeric. These foods include a varied range of nutrients and bioactive chemicals that aid in inflammation reduction, tissue healing, and overall wellness.

Note: Fruits and vegetables, whether eaten raw, cooked, or blended into smoothies, contain critical nutrients and phytochemicals that help reduce chronic inflammation and the risk of inflammatory disorders.

Whole Grains

Whole grains are an important part of an anti-inflammatory diet because of their high nutritional content, which includes fiber, vitamins, minerals, and phytonutrients. Unlike refined grains, which have lost their bran and germ during processing, whole grains retain all of the grain kernels, giving a variety of health benefits.

Including a variety of whole grains in your meals can help reduce chronic inflammation, promote digestive health, and boost overall well-being. Here's a closer look at the anti-inflammatory benefits of certain whole grains.

- **Oats:** Oats are a multipurpose whole grain that contains a lot of fiber, especially beta-glucan, a soluble fiber with anti-inflammatory qualities. Beta-glucan lowers cholesterol, stabilizes blood sugar, and promotes the growth of good bacteria, all of which improve gut health. Oats also include antioxidants, vitamins, and minerals, which aid in their anti-inflammatory properties.
- **Quinoa**: Quinoa is a gluten-free whole grain high in protein, fiber, vitamins, and minerals. It includes all nine necessary amino acids, making it an ideal protein source for vegetarians and vegans. Quinoa also contains phytonutrients such as flavonoids, saponins, and polyphenols, which are anti-inflammatory and antioxidant. Incorporating quinoa into salads, stir-fries, and grain bowls can help diversify the diet while also providing critical nutrients.
- **Brown Rice**: Brown rice is a complete grain that includes more fiber, vitamins, and minerals than white rice, which has had the bran and germ removed. Brown rice contains complex carbs, which are processed more slowly and assist in regulating blood sugar levels. It also contains phytonutrients including lignans and anti-inflammatory phenolic compounds. Using brown rice instead of white rice in meals can help reduce inflammation and enhance metabolic health.

- **Barley:** Barley is a nutritious whole grain high in fiber, specifically beta-glucan, which lowers cholesterol and improves digestive health. Barley also includes antioxidants including phenolic acids and flavonoids, which are anti-inflammatory. Consuming barley as a side dish, soup, stew, or salad can help boost fiber intake and enhance satiety.

- **Buckwheat**: Contrary to popular belief, buckwheat is a gluten-free pseudocereal high in protein, fiber, vitamins, and minerals rather than a true grain. Buckwheat includes rutin, a flavonoid that has anti-inflammatory and antioxidant effects that assist in reducing oxidative stress and inflammation. Buckwheat groats, flour, and noodles are common ingredients in a variety of culinary recipes.

- **Millet**: Millet is a gluten-free whole grain high in fiber, protein, vitamins, and minerals. It contains phytonutrients such as lignans, phenolic acids, and flavonoids, which are anti-inflammatory and antioxidant. Millet is a versatile grain that may be used to make porridge, salads, pilafs, and baked products, offering a nutrient-dense alternative to refined grains.

- **Whole Grain Bread and Pasta**: Choosing whole grain bread and pasta over refined alternatives is a simple way to get more whole grains into your diet. Look for products branded "100% whole grain" or "whole wheat" to get the most nutritional value. Whole grain bread and pasta include complex carbohydrates, fiber, and important nutrients that assist in reducing inflammation and promote overall health.

Nuts and Seeds

Nuts and seeds are nutrient-dense foods that contain healthful fats, protein, fiber, vitamins, minerals, and phytochemicals. Including a variety of nuts and seeds in your diet can help reduce chronic inflammation, promote heart health, and boost overall well-being. Let's take a closer look at the anti-inflammatory qualities of several nuts and seeds:

- **Almonds**: Almonds are a nutritional powerhouse, high in monounsaturated fats, protein, fiber, vitamin E, magnesium, and antioxidants. Almonds include flavonoids, phenolic acids, and other phytochemicals that are anti-inflammatory and antioxidant in nature. Regular eating of almonds has been linked to lower levels of inflammatory markers and better cardiovascular health

- **Walnuts:** Walnuts contain alpha-linolenic acid (ALA), an omega-3 fatty acid that has anti-inflammatory properties. In addition to ALA, walnuts contain polyphenols, vitamin E, and other antioxidants that assist in preventing oxidative stress and inflammation. Walnuts have been found to improve lipid profiles, reduce inflammation, and minimize the risk of chronic diseases.

- **Flaxseeds**: Flaxseeds are one of the highest plant sources of ALA, making them an important component of an anti-inflammatory diet. Flaxseeds include lignans, which are antioxidants and anti-inflammatory. Ground flaxseeds can be included in smoothies, yogurt, cereal, and baked products to increase omega-3 intake and improve heart health.

- **Chia Seeds**: Chia seeds are another high-quality source of ALA and fiber, making a nutritious supplement to any diet. Chia seeds include antioxidants such as quercetin, caffeic acid, and chlorogenic acid, which assist in reducing inflammation and oxidative stress. Adding chia seeds to beverages, puddings, salads, and baked goods can help you get more nutrients and feel fuller for longer.

- **Pumpkin Seeds**: Pumpkin seeds, often called pepitas, are high in protein, fiber, vitamins, minerals, and antioxidants. Pumpkin seeds include zinc, magnesium, and omega-3 fatty acids, all of which serve to regulate immunological function and prevent inflammation. Roasted pumpkin seeds are a tasty and nutritious snack, or they may be mixed into salads, soups, and trail mixes to add crunch and flavor.

- **Sunflower Seeds**: Sunflower seeds include vitamin E, an antioxidant that reduces inflammation and protects against oxidative damage. Sunflower seeds also include selenium, magnesium, and other minerals that promote immunological and cardiovascular health. Sunflower seeds make a great snack or can be sprinkled on salads, yogurt, or oatmeal for extra nourishment.

- **Sesame Seeds**: Sesame seeds are high in lignans, antioxidants, and anti-inflammatory chemicals, which assist in reducing inflammation and promote heart health. Sesame seeds include calcium, magnesium, and other elements that promote bone health and overall well-being.

Toasted sesame seeds can be used as a garnish in savory dishes, salads, and stir-fries, or mashed into tahini paste to make sauces and dressings.

Herbs and Spices

Herbs and spices have been used for generations to enhance the flavor and scent of dishes, as well as for their medical effects. Many herbs and spices include bioactive chemicals that have strong anti-inflammatory and antioxidant properties. Including a variety of herbs and spices in your diet can help reduce chronic inflammation, boost immunological function, and improve overall health. Below are some herbs and spices with anti-inflammatory properties:

- **Turmeric:** Turmeric includes curcumin, a bioactive molecule that has strong anti-inflammatory and antioxidant properties. Curcumin has been extensively explored for its ability to suppress inflammatory pathways, reduce oxidative stress, and regulate immunological responses. Consuming turmeric or curcumin supplements has been found to help with the symptoms of inflammatory illnesses such as arthritis, inflammatory bowel disease, and metabolic syndrome.
- **Ginger**: Ginger includes gingerol, a bioactive molecule that has anti-inflammatory and pain-relieving qualities. Gingerol suppresses inflammatory enzymes and pathways, which reduces inflammation and pain in illnesses including osteoarthritis and rheumatoid arthritis.

Ginger, whether consumed as a drink, spice, or supplement, can help relieve nausea, indigestion, and inflammation.

- **Cinnamon**: Cinnamon includes cinnamaldehyde and other polyphenols that have anti-inflammatory and antioxidant properties. Cinnamon reduces inflammation, lowers blood sugar levels, and boosts insulin sensitivity in people with diabetes and metabolic syndrome. Adding cinnamon to breakfast, smoothies, baked products, and savory dishes can improve flavor while also providing health advantages.

- **Garlic:** Garlic contains allicin, a sulfur molecule that has anti-inflammatory and immune-boosting qualities. Allicin suppresses inflammatory enzymes and pathways, which lowers inflammation and oxidative stress in the body. Consuming garlic regularly has been linked to lower levels of inflammatory markers and a lower risk of chronic diseases like cardiovascular disease and cancer.

- **Rosemary**: Rosemary includes rosmarinic acid and other polyphenols that are anti-inflammatory and antioxidant. Rosemary reduces inflammation, protects against oxidative stress, and enhances cognitive function. Adding fresh or dried rosemary to marinades, sauces, roasted vegetables, and meat meals can boost flavor while also providing health advantages.

- **Cayenne Pepper**: Cayenne pepper contains capsaicin, which has analgesic and anti-inflammatory properties. Capsaicin blocks pain receptors and inflammatory pathways, lowering pain and inflammation caused by illnesses including arthritis and neuropathy.

Cayenne pepper can enhance the flavor and intensity of foods while also delivering health benefits.

> **Cloves**: Cloves contain eugenol, which has anti-inflammatory and analgesic qualities. Eugenol reduces inflammation, relieves pain, and inhibits inflammatory enzymes and pathways. Using whole or ground cloves in foods, drinks, and baked goods can improve flavor and provide health benefits.

> **Black Pepper**: Black pepper includes piperine, which increases the bioavailability of other minerals and phytochemicals. Piperine has anti-inflammatory and antioxidant effects, which assist in reducing inflammation and improve digestion. Including black pepper in savory foods, salads, and soups can improve flavor and nutrient absorption.

Legumes and Beans

Legumes and beans are nutrient-dense foods that play an important part in an anti-inflammatory diet due to their high fiber, protein, vitamins, minerals, and phytonutrients. Including a variety of legumes and beans in your meals can help reduce chronic inflammation, improve digestive health, and promote overall well-being. Below are some anti-inflammatory benefits of various legumes and beans.

> **Lentils**: Lentils are a multipurpose legume that contains fiber, protein, folate, iron, and other important nutrients. Lentils include soluble fiber, which helps balance blood sugar levels, induce satiety, and support digestive health.

Lentils include polyphenols, flavonoids, and other phytochemicals that have anti-inflammatory and antioxidant activities.

▸ **Chickpeas (Garbanzo Beans):** Chickpeas are a staple legume in many cuisines, high in fiber, protein, vitamins, minerals, and antioxidants. Chickpeas include both soluble and insoluble fiber, which promotes regular bowel motions, lowers cholesterol and reduces inflammation. Regular consumption of chickpeas has been linked to improved glycemic control, weight management, and cardiovascular health.

▸ **Black Beans:** Black beans are nutrient-dense legumes high in fiber, protein, folate, magnesium, and antioxidants. The soluble fiber in black beans lowers cholesterol, stabilizes blood sugar, and promotes gut health. Black beans contain anthocyanins, flavonoids, and other phytochemicals with anti-inflammatory and antioxidant properties.

▸ **Kidney Beans:** Kidney beans are a great source of plant protein, fiber, vitamins, and minerals. Kidney beans include resistant starch, a fiber that acts as a prebiotic, feeding good bacteria in the gut and improving digestive health. Regular consumption of kidney beans can help reduce inflammation, control cholesterol, and assist weight management.

▸ **Pinto Beans:** Pinto beans are a multipurpose legume high in fiber, protein, folate, and antioxidants that are popular in Mexican and Southwestern cuisine. Pinto beans include polyphenols, flavonoids, and other phytochemicals that assist in reducing inflammation, protect against oxidative stress, and promote heart health.

Pinto beans can be used in soups, stews, salads, and chili to give critical nutrients while also increasing satiety.

- **Green Peas**: Green peas are a healthy legume high in fiber, protein, vitamins, and minerals. Green peas contain antioxidants such as flavonoids, carotenoids, and polyphenols, which assist in preventing inflammation and oxidative stress. Green peas can assist improve digestive health, lower cholesterol, and lower the risk of chronic diseases.
- **Lima Beans**: Lima beans, often called butter beans, are a creamy and nutritious legume high in fiber, protein, folate, and potassium. Lima beans include soluble fiber, which aids in blood sugar regulation, satiety, and digestive health. Lima beans also contain phytochemicals called saponins and flavonoids, which have anti-inflammatory and antioxidant benefits.

Fatty Fish and Omega-3 Fatty Acids

Fatty fish and omega-3 fatty acids are critical components of an anti-inflammatory diet due to their powerful anti-inflammatory and heart-healthy qualities. Omega-3 fatty acids, particularly eicosapentaenoic acid (EPA) and docosahexaenoic acid (DHA) are polyunsaturated fats that play key roles in lowering inflammation, maintaining cardiovascular health, and promoting overall well-being. Let's take a closer look at some benefits of fatty fish and omega-3s.

- **Fatty Fish**: Fatty fish such as salmon, mackerel, sardines, trout, herring, and tuna are good providers of omega-3 fatty acids, notably EPA and DHA. These fatty acids are absorbed into cell membranes and act as precursors to strong anti-inflammatory mediators known as resolvins and protectins. Consuming fatty fish regularly can help reduce systemic inflammation, lower inflammatory markers, and minimize the risk of inflammatory illnesses.

- **EPA and DHA:** EPA and DHA are long-chain omega-3 fatty acids found primarily in fatty fish and seafood. These fatty acids have anti-inflammatory, anti-thrombotic, and anti-arrhythmic properties, which help reduce inflammation, prevent blood clot formation, and regulate heart rhythm. EPA and DHA also promote brain health, cognitive function, and mood management, making them important nutrients for overall health.

- **Alpha-Linolenic Acid (ALA):** Alpha-linolenic acid (ALA) is a plant-derived omega-3 fatty acid found in walnuts, flaxseeds, chia seeds, hemp seeds, and soybeans. ALA can be transformed into EPA and DHA in the body, however the conversion rate is modest. Consuming foods high in ALA can still give some anti-inflammatory benefits and improve cardiovascular health, especially for those who follow a plant-based diet.

Anti-Inflammatory Effects: Omega-3 fatty acids reduce inflammation by reducing the production of pro-inflammatory eicosanoids, cytokines, and adhesion molecules and increasing the synthesis of anti-inflammatory mediators.

EPA and DHA compete with arachidonic acid (AA) for incorporation into cell membranes and act as substrates for the formation of anti-inflammatory eicosanoids. Omega-3 fatty acids prevent chronic inflammation by modifying inflammatory pathways and lowering the risk of inflammatory disorders such as cardiovascular disease, rheumatoid arthritis, and inflammatory bowel disease.

Cardiovascular Health: Omega-3 fatty acids have been extensively researched for their cardiovascular benefits, which include lower triglyceride levels, lower blood pressure, improved endothelial function, and a lower risk of atherosclerosis and cardiovascular disease. Regular eating of fatty fish or omega-3 supplements has been linked to improved lipid profiles, lower inflammation, and better vascular health.

Brain Health: DHA is a crucial structural component of brain cell membranes, making it especially vital for brain health and cognitive function. Adequate DHA intake during pregnancy and infancy is necessary for fetal brain development and cognitive function. Omega-3 fatty acids have neuroprotective properties and may lower the risk of neurodegenerative illnesses including Alzheimer's and Parkinson's.

Consuming fatty fish at least twice a week, as well as plant-based omega-3 sources, will assist in ensuring an appropriate intake of these critical fatty acids while also supporting overall health and well-being. Individuals who may struggle to satisfy their omega-3 needs through diet alone may also consider omega-3 supplements produced from fish oil, krill oil, or algal oil.

CHAPTER 3: FOODS TO AVOID OR LIMIT

We will look at foods that can cause inflammation and aggravate existing diseases. Individuals who limit or avoid these foods can better manage chronic inflammation and improve overall health. Here are some essential food groups to consider.

Processed and Fried Foods

Processed and fried meals are key causes of chronic inflammation because they contain high levels of harmful fats, processed carbs, chemicals, and preservatives. Regular use of these foods can cause oxidative stress, insulin resistance, dysbiosis (an imbalance of gut bacteria), and systemic inflammation.

- **Trans Fats**: Trans fats are commonly found in processed and fried foods. They are formed during the hydrogenation process used to solidify liquid oils. Trans fats elevate LDL (bad) cholesterol while decreasing HDL (good) cholesterol, which contributes to inflammation, oxidative stress, and heart disease. Fried meals, baked products, margarine, and processed snacks such as chips and crackers are common sources of trans fat.
- **Unhealthy Cooking Oils:** Fried foods are often prepared using unhealthy oils such as vegetable oil, corn oil, soybean oil, and canola oil, which are high in omega-6 fatty acids and prone to oxidation.

Excessive consumption of these oils can disturb the body's omega-3 and omega-6 fatty acid balance, causing inflammation and increasing the risk of chronic diseases. The repeated heating of these oils during frying might develop hazardous substances known as advanced glycation end products (AGEs), which increase inflammation and oxidative stress.

- **Additives and Preservatives**: Processed foods frequently contain additives, preservatives, taste enhancers, colorings, and artificial sweeteners, which can cause immunological reactions and inflammation. Common additives, such as monosodium glutamate (MSG), high-fructose corn syrup (HFCS), artificial food colors, and sodium nitrate preservatives, have been related to inflammation, allergic reactions, and other health problems.

- **High Sodium Content**: Processed and fried foods are high in sodium, which can lead to inflammation, water retention, and high blood pressure. High salt intake has been linked to an increased risk of hypertension, cardiovascular disease, and renal damage. Consuming processed meals in moderation and choosing lower-sodium alternatives can help minimize salt consumption and its inflammatory consequences.

- **Nutrient Deficiency**: Processed and fried meals frequently lack key nutrients such as vitamins, minerals, fiber, and antioxidants, all of which are necessary for inflammation reduction and overall health. Instead, they deliver empty calories that lack nutritional value, resulting in vitamin shortages and chronic inflammation.

Choosing natural, minimally processed foods high in nutrients can help reduce inflammation and support overall health.

Refined Carbohydrates and Their Role in Inflammation

Refined carbohydrates are highly processed grains that have lost their fiber, vitamins, minerals, and phytonutrients during milling and manufacture. These highly processed carbohydrates have a high glycemic index, resulting in rapid blood sugar increases, increased insulin release, and metabolic disruptions. Regular use of refined carbs has been related to inflammation, insulin resistance, and an increased risk of chronic diseases like type 2 diabetes, heart disease, and obesity. Let's take a closer look at the inflammatory effects of refined carbohydrates:

- High Glycemic Index: Refined carbohydrates such as white bread, white rice, pasta, pastries, and sugary snacks have a high glycemic index, resulting in a quick rise in blood glucose levels following ingestion. This quick increase in blood sugar causes the pancreas to secrete more insulin, which helps transport glucose into cells for energy or storage. Chronic consumption of high-glycemic meals can cause insulin resistance, in which cells become less receptive to insulin's activities, resulting in inflammation and metabolic malfunction.

- Insulin Resistance: Insulin resistance develops when cells in the body lose sensitivity to the effects of insulin, resulting in decreased glucose absorption and utilization.

As a result, the pancreas generates more insulin to compensate for the resistance, which raises insulin levels in the bloodstream. High insulin levels can cause inflammation by activating inflammatory pathways and boosting the production of pro-inflammatory cytokines. Insulin resistance is a defining feature of metabolic syndrome and is strongly linked to chronic inflammation and the development of type 2 diabetes.

- Promotion of Adiposity: Refined carbs are frequently lacking in fiber and nutrients but high in calories, resulting in excessive calorie consumption and weight gain. Excess body fat, especially visceral fat around the abdomen, is a key source of pro-inflammatory cytokines and adipokines, all of which lead to chronic inflammation. Consumption of refined carbs has been associated with increased adiposity and abdominal obesity, which worsens inflammation and metabolic dysfunction.

- Dysbiosis: Refined carbohydrates increase the proliferation of pro-inflammatory gut bacteria while inhibiting beneficial bacteria, resulting in gut dysbiosis (microbial imbalance). Dysbiosis is related to increased intestinal permeability (leaky gut), which allows bacterial endotoxins into the circulation and causes systemic inflammation. Chronic inflammation caused by dysbiosis can lead to a variety of inflammatory illnesses, including inflammatory bowel disease, autoimmune diseases, and metabolic abnormalities.

> Oxidative Stress: Refined carbohydrates contribute to oxidative stress and the creation of reactive oxygen species (ROS) via a variety of mechanisms, including enhanced glycation (the binding of sugar molecules to proteins) and advanced glycation end product (AGE) development. Oxidative stress harms cells, tissues, and DNA, causing inflammatory reactions and contributing to the onset of chronic illnesses. Antioxidants present in whole, minimally processed meals can help lower oxidative stress and inflammation.

Red and Processed Meats

Red and processed meats have been related to inflammation and an increased risk of chronic diseases like heart disease, cancer, and diabetes. These meats contain saturated fats, cholesterol, and chemicals produced during processing that can cause inflammation and oxidative stress in the body. Let's take a closer look at the inflammatory consequences of red and processed meats.

> Saturated Fats: Red meats like beef, lamb, and hog are high in saturated fats, which have been linked to elevated levels of inflammatory markers in the bloodstream. Saturated fats can trigger inflammatory pathways in the body, resulting in chronic low-grade inflammation. Excessive consumption of saturated fat has been linked to insulin resistance, endothelial dysfunction, and an increased risk of cardiovascular disease.

- Advanced Glycation End Products (AGEs): Processed meats, such as bacon, sausage, hot dogs, and deli meats, can develop advanced glycation end products (AGEs) when cooked using methods such as smoking, curing, or grilling. AGEs are chemicals generated when sugars react with proteins or lipids during high-temperature cooking. Consumption of AGEs has been associated with increased oxidative stress, inflammation, and endothelial dysfunction, which all contribute to the development of chronic illnesses.

- Heme Iron: Red meat contains heme iron, a kind of iron found in animal tissues that can lead to oxidative stress and inflammation in the body. A high consumption of heme iron has been linked to an increased risk of colon cancer, cardiovascular disease, and other inflammatory disorders. The International Agency for Research on Cancer (IARC) has classed processed meats as carcinogenic to humans, citing their high heme iron concentration and the creation of carcinogenic chemicals during processing.

- Nitrates and Nitrites: Processed meats frequently contain nitrates and nitrites, which serve as preservatives and color enhancers. Nitrates and nitrites can combine during digestion to generate nitrosamines, which are strong carcinogens that can damage DNA and cause inflammation. Regular eating of processed meats has been related to an increased risk of colorectal, stomach, and other cancers.

- Trimethylamine N-Oxide (TMAO): Red meats are abundant in carnitine and choline, which can be processed by gut bacteria into trimethylamine (TMA) and then transformed into trimethylamine N-oxide (TMAO) in the liver.

High levels of TMAO have been linked to an increased risk of cardiovascular disease and inflammation. Consumption of red meat, especially when cooked at high temperatures, might increase the synthesis of TMAO, contributing to chronic inflammation and cardiovascular risk.

- Pro-inflammatory Compounds: Red and processed meats include pro-inflammatory compounds such as arachidonic acid, a precursor to inflammatory eicosanoids. Animal fats include significant quantities of arachidonic acid, which can contribute to inflammation when taken in excess. Furthermore, the presence of heterocyclic amines (HCAs) and polycyclic aromatic hydrocarbons (PAHs) in charred or grilled meats can worsen inflammation and raise cancer risk.

Dairy Products and Their Effect on Inflammation

Dairy products, such as milk, cheese, yogurt, and butter, have been debated for their potential effects on inflammation and health. While dairy products are high in critical nutrients such as calcium, protein, and vitamins, they also include saturated fats and some proteins, which may cause inflammation in certain people. Let's take a closer look at the link between dairy products and inflammation:

Saturated Fats: Many dairy products, particularly full-fat options such as whole milk, cheese, and butter, contain high levels of saturated fat. A high consumption of saturated fats has been linked to higher levels of inflammatory markers and an increased risk of cardiovascular disease.

However, it is important to note that not all saturated fats are the same, and some dairy products, such as yogurt and some cheeses, may have a neutral or even favorable effect on inflammation due to their particular nutrient profile.

<u>Pro-inflammatory Proteins</u>: Some people have reported that dairy proteins, notably casein and whey, have pro-inflammatory qualities. Casein, in particular, has been linked to immunological responses and inflammatory disorders such as acne and eczema in sensitive individuals. Whey protein, on the other hand, may have both anti-inflammatory and pro-inflammatory properties, depending on the processing method and individual tolerance.

<u>Lactose Intolerance:</u> Lactose intolerance, or the inability to digest lactose (the sugar contained in milk), can cause gastrointestinal symptoms such as bloating, gas, diarrhea, and stomach discomfort. While lactose intolerance is not directly connected to inflammation, the symptoms can cause gut irritation and discomfort, perhaps exacerbating pre-existing inflammatory diseases in some people.

<u>Bioactive components</u>: Dairy products include bioactive components such as peptides, lipids, and minerals, which have anti-inflammatory properties. In animal and human research, bioactive peptides generated from milk proteins have been found to alter immune responses and exert anti-inflammatory effects. Dairy-derived calcium and vitamin D may also have immune-regulating effects that could help reduce inflammation.

<u>Fermented Dairy Products</u>: Fermented dairy products such as yogurt and kefir contain probiotics, which are helpful bacteria that have been found to improve gut health and immunological function. Probiotics may help to reduce inflammation by encouraging the growth of good gut bacteria while reducing the growth of pathogens. Furthermore, fermentation may increase the bioavailability of some minerals while decreasing lactose content, making fermented dairy products more palatable for people who are lactose intolerant.

<u>Individual Variability</u>: It is critical to understand that individual responses to dairy products can vary greatly depending on genetics, gut microbiota composition, and underlying health issues. While some people experience inflammation or gastrointestinal discomfort when they consume dairy, others tolerate it well and gain nutrition from it.

Alcohol's Impact on Inflammation

Alcohol use has been linked to both pro-inflammatory and anti-inflammatory effects, depending on criteria such as quantity drank, frequency ingested, individual genetics, and general health status. While moderate alcohol consumption may have certain health benefits, excessive or persistent drinking can cause inflammation, oxidative stress, and an increased risk of inflammatory illnesses. Let's take a closer look at the association between alcohol and inflammation:

▷ <u>Pro-inflammatory Effects</u>: Excessive alcohol consumption can cause inflammation via a variety of methods. Alcohol metabolism generates reactive oxygen species (ROS) and other harmful byproducts, which cause oxidative stress and tissue damage. Chronic alcohol intake can also alter gut barrier function, allowing bacterial endotoxins into the bloodstream and causing systemic inflammation. Furthermore, alcohol can activate inflammatory pathways in immune cells, resulting in the release of pro-inflammatory cytokines and chemokines.

▷ <u>Liver Inflammation:</u> Chronic alcohol intake is a major cause of alcoholic liver disease, which is marked by inflammation, steatosis (fatty liver), fibrosis, and, eventually, cirrhosis. Several factors contribute to alcohol-induced liver inflammation, including oxidative stress, lipid peroxidation, mitochondrial dysfunction, and activation of inflammatory signaling pathways. Inflammatory cells invade the liver in reaction to alcohol-induced injury, causing chronic inflammation and tissue destruction.

▷ <u>Gut Microbiota Dysbiosis:</u> Alcohol can alter the composition and function of the gut microbiota, resulting in dysbiosis (microbial imbalance) and intestinal inflammation. Alcohol changes the intestinal ecology, encouraging the growth of harmful bacteria while lowering the population of helpful bacteria. Dysbiosis can cause increased intestinal permeability (leaky gut), which allows bacterial endotoxins to enter the bloodstream and cause immunological reactions and inflammation throughout the body.

- <u>Immunological Dysfunction:</u> Chronic alcohol consumption can compromise immunological function, leaving people more vulnerable to infections and inflammatory disorders. Alcohol inhibits the activity of immune cells such as macrophages, neutrophils, and lymphocytes, reducing their ability to fight infections and regulate inflammatory reactions. Chronic alcohol misuse is linked to an increased vulnerability to infections, poor wound healing, and dysregulated immunological responses.

- <u>Cardiovascular Inflammation</u>: Although moderate alcohol use has been linked to a lower risk of cardiovascular disease, excessive alcohol consumption can increase inflammation and oxidative stress in the cardiovascular system. Alcohol-induced inflammation can lead to endothelial dysfunction, arterial stiffness, atherosclerosis, and an elevated risk of cardiovascular events. Chronic alcohol usage is linked to hypertension, cardiomyopathy, and other inflammatory cardiovascular diseases.

- <u>Individual Variability:</u> It is critical to understand that individual responses to alcohol might differ depending on genetics, age, gender, overall health state, and drinking habits. While some people can handle moderate alcohol consumption without ill effects, others may be more vulnerable to the inflammatory and health effects of alcohol.

Overall, moderate alcohol intake may have some health benefits, notably for cardiovascular health, but excessive or chronic alcohol drinking might induce inflammation and raise the risk of inflammatory disorders. It is best to consume alcohol in moderation and within prescribed parameters.

CHAPTER 4: ANTI-INFLAMMATORY DIETARY PATTERNS

We will look at different dietary methods that have been proven to lower inflammation and improve general health and well-being. These dietary patterns prioritize full, nutrient-dense foods high in antioxidants, phytonutrients, and anti-inflammatory components while limiting or eliminating pro-inflammatory foods. Here are some important anti-inflammatory eating habits.

Mediterranean Diet's

The Mediterranean diet is based on the traditional eating habits of countries bordering the Mediterranean Sea, including Greece, Italy, Spain, and southern France. It is well-known for its health benefits, including its capacity to reduce inflammation and lower the risk of chronic diseases. Here's a closer look at the essential components of the Mediterranean diet and their anti-inflammatory properties:

➤ Emphasis on Plant-Based Foods: The Mediterranean diet emphasizes eating a wide variety of plant-based foods, such as fruits, vegetables, whole grains, legumes, nuts, seeds, and olive oil. These plant-based foods are high in antioxidants, vitamins, minerals, and phytonutrients, which have strong anti-inflammatory qualities. The Mediterranean diet's high intake of plant-based foods reduces oxidative stress and inflammation in the body.

- <u>Healthy Fats</u>: The Mediterranean diet contains healthy fats, particularly from olive oil, fatty fish, nuts, and seeds. Olive oil, in particular, is a staple of the Mediterranean diet and contains monounsaturated fats, particularly oleic acid, which has anti-inflammatory properties. Fatty fish such as salmon, mackerel, and sardines contain omega-3 fatty acids, which have been found to reduce inflammation and the risk of cardiovascular disease.

- <u>Modest Consumption of Dairy and Poultry</u>: The Mediterranean diet contains modest amounts of dairy products like yogurt and cheese, as well as lean poultry and eggs. While animal-derived meals are taken in smaller quantities than plant-based foods, they nonetheless include essential elements such as protein, calcium, and vitamin D. Choosing low-fat or reduced-fat dairy products can assist in lowering saturated fat intake and improve cardiovascular health.

- <u>Reduced Red Meat and Processed Foods</u>: The Mediterranean diet recommends minimizing red meat and processed foods, which are high in saturated fats, cholesterol, and pro-inflammatory chemicals. Instead, it focuses on lean protein sources such as poultry, fish, lentils, and plant-based protein substitutes. Reduced consumption of red meat and processed foods reduces inflammation, improves lipid profiles, and lowers the risk of chronic diseases such as cardiovascular disease and cancer.

- <u>Wine in Moderation:</u> The Mediterranean diet includes moderate consumption of red wine, especially when it is drunk with meals.

Red wine includes polyphenols, including resveratrol, which have antioxidant and anti-inflammatory properties. To minimize adverse health effects, alcohol should be consumed in moderation and within suggested limits.

‣ <u>Social and Lifestyle Factors:</u> In addition to nutritional choices, the Mediterranean lifestyle stresses social and cultural components of eating, such as sharing meals with family and friends, taking time to savor food, and engaging in regular physical activity. These lifestyle variables improve general health and may boost the Mediterranean diet's anti-inflammatory advantages.

The DASH Diet's Anti-Inflammatory

The Dietary Approaches to Stop Hypertension (DASH) diet is a well-studied dietary pattern that aims to lower blood pressure and minimize the risk of hypertension. While the DASH diet is primarily concerned with enhancing heart health, it also contains anti-inflammatory properties due to its concentration of full, nutrient-dense foods and the potential to promote overall metabolic health. Here's a closer look at the essential components of the DASH diet and their anti-inflammatory properties:

‣ <u>Rich in Fruits and Vegetables:</u> The DASH diet promotes the eating of a wide range of fruits and vegetables, which are high in antioxidants, vitamins, minerals, and phytonutrients. These plant-based meals have strong anti-inflammatory qualities, which assist in reducing oxidative stress and inflammation in the body.

Individuals who consume a variety of colored fruits and vegetables can support immunological function, reduce inflammation, and lessen their risk of chronic diseases.

▹ <u>High in Fiber:</u> The DASH diet has a lot of dietary fiber, which comes mostly from fruits and vegetables, whole grains, legumes, nuts, and seeds. Fiber promotes digestive health, regulates blood sugar levels, and reduces inflammation. Soluble fiber, in particular, has been demonstrated to alter immunological responses and reduce pro-inflammatory indicators in the body. Individuals can improve gut health, boost satiety, and reduce inflammation by eating a variety of fiber-rich meals.

▹ <u>Low in salt:</u> The DASH diet focuses on lowering salt intake to help lower blood pressure and reduce the risk of hypertension. Excessive sodium consumption can cause water retention, high blood pressure, and inflammation in the body. Individuals can reduce inflammation and improve cardiovascular health by avoiding high-sodium foods such as processed meats, canned soups, salty snacks, and fast food. Instead, the DASH diet promotes the use of herbs, spices, and other flavorings to improve the taste of meals without the need for extra salt.

▹ <u>Moderate Lean Protein:</u> The DASH diet contains moderate amounts of lean protein from poultry, fish, legumes, nuts, and seeds. These protein-rich meals supply vital amino acids for muscle repair and growth while containing less saturated fat than red meat and processed meats.

Individuals can reduce inflammation, improve lipid profiles, and support general metabolic health by consuming lean protein sources as well as plant-based proteins like legumes and nuts.

▷ <u>Healthy Fats</u>: Unlike the Mediterranean diet, which emphasizes healthy fats, the DASH diet advocates the consumption of unsaturated fats over saturated and trans fats. Unsaturated fats, such as olive oil, avocados, almonds, and fatty fish, have anti-inflammatory qualities and can help lower the risk of cardiovascular disease. Individuals can reduce inflammation and improve heart health by focusing on good fats and limiting their consumption of saturated and trans fats.

▷ <u>Overall Nutrient Density</u>: The DASH diet emphasizes nutrient-dense foods that provide critical vitamins, minerals, and antioxidants. The DASH diet, which emphasizes whole, minimally processed foods such as fruits, vegetables, whole grains, lean meats, and healthy fats, helps to guarantee optimal nutrient intake for lowering inflammation, boosting immune function, and improving general health and well-being.

Vegetarian and Vegan

Let's take a closer look at vegetarian and vegan diets, including their major components, health benefits, and potential drawbacks:

Vegetarian and vegan diets can be naturally anti-inflammatory since they emphasize entire, plant-based meals high in antioxidants, fiber, vitamins, minerals, and phytonutrients. These diets have been linked to decreased inflammation, better metabolic health, and a lower risk of chronic diseases like heart disease, type 2 diabetes, and some malignancies. Here's how vegetarian and vegan diets support an anti-inflammatory eating pattern:

Vegetarian Diet

▹ <u>Plant-Based Foods</u>: Vegetarian diets focus on plant-based foods such as fruits, vegetables, whole grains, legumes, nuts, seeds, and plant-derived oils. These foods are high in fiber, vitamins, minerals, and phytonutrients, which help with general health and well-being.

▹ <u>Variety of Protein Sources</u>: Vegetarian diets eliminate meat, poultry, and seafood but contain a variety of protein sources such as legumes (beans, lentils, chickpeas), tofu, tcmpeh, edamame, seitan, nuts, seeds, and dairy products (for lacto vegetarians). These protein sources contain the essential amino acids required for muscle regeneration, immunological function, and overall health.

▹ <u>Dairy and Eggs</u>: The vegetarian diet can contain dairy products (lacto-vegetarian) and eggs (ovo-vegetarian). These animal-derived meals contain additional protein, calcium, vitamin D, and other minerals. Including dairy and eggs in your diet can help you achieve your nutritional needs and get enough vitamins and minerals.

▷ <u>Flexibility and Adaptability</u>: Vegetarian diets are flexible and adaptable to personal tastes and dietary constraints. There are several forms of vegetarian diets, including lacto-vegetarian, ovo-vegetarian, lacto-ovo-vegetarian (which includes dairy and eggs), and pescatarian. Individuals can tailor their vegetarian diet to meet their particular preferences, cultural influences, and nutritional requirements.

▷ <u>Health Benefits</u>: Vegetarian diets have been linked to a variety of health benefits, including a lower risk of chronic diseases such as heart disease, hypertension, type 2 diabetes, specific malignancies, and obesity. A diet rich in fruits, vegetables, whole grains, and legumes contains antioxidants, fiber, and other bioactive elements that assist in reducing inflammation, support gut health, and improve metabolic function.

Vegan diet

▷ <u>Plant-Based Exclusivity</u>: Vegan diets do not include any animal-derived items, such as meat, poultry, seafood, dairy products, eggs, or honey. They concentrate solely on plant-based foods, including fruits, vegetables, whole grains, legumes, nuts, seeds, and plant-derived oils.

▷ <u>Plant-Based Protein Sources</u>: Vegan diets rely on plant-based proteins to meet protein requirements, such as legumes, tofu, tempeh, seitan, edamame, nuts, seeds, and plant-based protein powders.

These protein sources contain the essential amino acids required for muscle regeneration, immunological function, and overall health.

▷ <u>Nutrient Considerations</u>: While vegan diets can be nutrient-dense, some nutrients, such as vitamin B12, iron, calcium, vitamin D, omega-3 fatty acids, and zinc, may require extra care. Fortified meals, supplements, and smart food choices can all contribute to optimal nutrient consumption. Fortified plant kinds of milk, tofu, walnuts, and leafy greens are examples of plant-based calcium sources, whereas fortified foods and supplements can provide vitamin B12.

▷ <u>Environmental and Ethical issues</u>: Vegan diets are frequently driven by concerns about animal welfare, environmental sustainability, and ethical issues. Individuals who forgo animal products lessen their environmental impact, save natural resources, and protect animals. Vegan diets promote the values of compassion, sustainability, and environmental care.

▷ <u>Health Benefits</u>: Vegan diets have been linked to a variety of health benefits, including lower risk of chronic diseases like heart disease, hypertension, type 2 diabetes, certain malignancies, and obesity. A diet rich in plant-based foods contains antioxidants, fiber, vitamins, minerals, and phytonutrients, all of which assist in reducing inflammation, support gut health, and improve metabolic function.

Paleo

The Paleo diet, also known as the Paleolithic diet or the caveman diet, is based on our prehistoric predecessors' assumed nutritional habits during the Paleolithic period. While the Paleo diet focuses on foods available to hunter-gatherers, it also adheres to several anti-inflammatory dietary guidelines. Here's a closer look at the Paleo diet and anti-inflammatory eating:

- <u>Emphasis on entire, Unprocessed Foods:</u> The Paleo diet focuses on eating entire, unprocessed foods including fruits, vegetables, nuts, seeds, lean meats, and seafood. The Paleo diet promotes general health and well-being by putting nutrient-dense foods first over processed and refined meals.

- <u>High in Fruits and Vegetables:</u> Fruits and vegetables are vital components of the Paleo diet, supplying vitamins, minerals, antioxidants, and phytonutrients. These plant-based foods assist to reduce inflammation, improve immunological function, and minimize the risk of chronic disease. The Paleo diet, which emphasizes a variety of colorful fruits and vegetables, ensures a broad intake of nutrients that contribute to general wellness.

- <u>Healthy Fats:</u> Avocados, nuts, seeds, and plant-derived oils such as olive and coconut oil are all sources of healthy fats on the Paleo diet. These fats contain important fatty acids, such as omega-3 and omega-6 fatty acids, which have anti-inflammatory characteristics and assist in reducing inflammation in the body. By integrating healthy fats into meals, the Paleo diet promotes cardiovascular health and overall well-being.

- <u>Lean Protein Sources</u>: The Paleo diet contains lean protein sources such as poultry, fish, and grass-fed meats. These protein sources contain the essential amino acids required for muscle regeneration, immunological function, and overall health. The Paleo diet promotes muscular health and decreases inflammation by focusing on lean protein sources and limiting the consumption of processed meats and high-fat meat cuts.

- <u>Processed Food Elimination</u>: The Paleo diet does not include processed or refined foods such as sugar, refined grains, artificial additives, or processed vegetable oils. These foods have been associated with increased inflammation, insulin resistance, and chronic illnesses. The Paleo diet, which eliminates processed meals in favor of whole, nutrient-dense foods, helps to reduce inflammation, regulate blood sugar levels, and promote metabolic health.

- <u>Potential Reduction in Dairy and Grains</u>: While some Paleo diet versions recommend consuming dairy products and some grains in moderation, others urge for their elimination. Dairy and grains include components that might cause inflammation and digestive problems in some people, especially those who are lactose intolerant or gluten-sensitive. The Paleo diet, which limits or eliminates dairy and wheat, may help reduce inflammation and improve gut health in vulnerable individuals.

CHAPTER 5: MEAL PLANNING AND RECIPES

In the Meal Planning and Recipes chapter, we'll look at how to prepare nutritious, balanced meals that support anti-inflammatory eating habits. We'll also present a range of delectable recipes that use full, nutrient-dense foods to reduce inflammation and enhance general health and well-being. Whether you're following a certain dietary pattern, such as the Mediterranean diet, DASH diet, vegetarian, vegan, or Paleo diet, or just want to incorporate more anti-inflammatory items into your meals, we'll provide practical meal planning and cooking ideas. Let's get started by defining the fundamental components of efficient meal planning, followed by some great dishes to try at home.

Key Elements of Successful Meal Planning:

1. <u>Plan your Goals:</u> Before you begin meal planning, you should first determine your health and nutrition goals. Whether you want to reduce inflammation, lose weight, boost your energy, or simply consume more nutritious foods, knowing your goals will help you plan your meals.

2. <u>Understanding Your Dietary Preferences and Requirements</u>: Consider your dietary preferences, limits, or requirements, such as vegetarianism, veganism, gluten-free, dairy-free, or food allergies. Customize your meal plan to accommodate your preferences and satisfy your nutritional requirements.

3. <u>Make a weekly meal plan</u>: Plan your weekly meals, including breakfast, lunch, dinner, and snacks. Consider your schedule, available cooking time, and any impending events or activities that may affect your meal planning. Incorporate a variety and balance of fruits, vegetables, whole grains, lean meats, and healthy fats into your meals.

4. <u>Create Balanced Meals</u>: Each meal should have a healthy mix of macronutrients (carbohydrates, protein, and fat) and micronutrients (vitamins and minerals). Fill your plate with colorful fruits and vegetables, whole grains like quinoa or brown rice, lean meats like chicken, fish, tofu, or lentils, and healthy fats like avocado, almonds, and olive oil.

5. <u>Use Seasonal and Local Ingredients</u>: When preparing your meals, make sure to include seasonal food and local ingredients. Seasonal foods are not only fresher and more tasty, but they are also less expensive and more environmentally friendly. To get fresh, local products, go to farmer's markets or join a community-supported agriculture (CSA) program.

6. <u>Plan ahead of time</u>: Save time during the week by preparing ingredients and meals ahead of time. Wash and chop fruits and veggies, boil grains and meats, and prepare snacks and ingredients for quick meals. Spending a little time on meal prep can make healthy eating more convenient and accessible throughout the week.

7. <u>Incorporate Variety and Flexibility</u>: Incorporate a diversity of flavors, textures, and cuisines to make your meals more fascinating and pleasurable.

To make your meals more fascinating, try new recipes, ingredients, and cooking methods. Allow for flexibility in your meal plan to account for schedule changes, unanticipated events, and spontaneous desires.

8. <u>Observe Portion Sizes</u>: To avoid overeating, use smaller plates and utensils, practice mindful eating, and pay attention to your body's hunger and fullness signs. Instead of overeating, eat until you're content, and strive for balance and moderation in your food choices.

9. <u>Be Organized and Stock Up on Staples</u>: Stock your cupboard, fridge, and freezer with everyday staples like nutritious grains, canned beans, herbs and spices, healthy oils, and frozen fruits and veggies. Keeping these necessities on hand makes meal planning and cooking easier and more effective.

10. <u>Be Flexible and Adapt as Needed</u>: Be adaptable and open to adjusting your meal plan in response to changes in circumstances, preferences, or nutritional requirements. If a recipe doesn't come out as planned or you're short on time, have basic salads, stir-fries, or grain bowls on hand for quick meals.

Recipes.

Breakfast Recipes.

Breakfast is often considered the most important meal of the day, providing energy and nutrients to kick-start your morning. Here are some delicious and nutritious breakfast recipes that incorporate anti-inflammatory ingredients and support overall health and well-being:

1. Berry Smoothie Bowl

Ingredients:

- 1 cup mixed berries (such as strawberries, blueberries, raspberries)
- 1 ripe banana
- 1/2 cup spinach or kale leaves
- 1/2 cup unsweetened almond milk or coconut water
- 1 tablespoon chia seeds
- Toppings: sliced banana, fresh berries, granola, shredded coconut, almond slices

Instructions:

- In a blender, combine the mixed berries, banana, spinach or kale, almond milk or coconut water, and chia seeds. Blend until smooth and creamy.
- Pour the smoothie into a bowl and top with sliced banana, fresh berries, granola, shredded coconut, and almond slices.

- Enjoy immediately as a refreshing and nutrient-packed breakfast.

2. Avocado Toast with Poached Egg

Ingredients:

- 2 slices whole-grain bread or gluten-free bread
- 1 ripe avocado
- 2 eggs
- Salt and pepper to taste
- Optional toppings: cherry tomatoes, microgreens, red pepper flakes

Instructions:

- Toast the bread slices until golden brown and crispy.
- Mash the ripe avocado in a bowl and season with salt and pepper to taste.
- In a pot of simmering water, gently crack the eggs and poach them until the whites are set but the yolks are still runny, about 3-4 minutes.
- Spread the mashed avocado evenly onto the toasted bread slices.
- Carefully place a poached egg on top of each avocado toast.
- Garnish with optional toppings such as sliced cherry tomatoes, microgreens, or red pepper flakes.
- Serve immediately for a satisfying and protein-rich breakfast.

3. Turmeric Chia Pudding

Ingredients:

- 1/4 cup chia seeds
- 1 cup unsweetened almond milk or coconut milk
- 1/2 teaspoon ground turmeric
- 1/2 teaspoon ground cinnamon
- 1 tablespoon maple syrup or honey (optional)
- Toppings: sliced banana, berries, chopped nuts, shredded coconut

Instructions:

- In a bowl or jar, combine the chia seeds, almond milk or coconut milk, ground turmeric, ground cinnamon, and maple syrup or honey (if using). Stir well to combine.
- Cover the bowl or jar and refrigerate for at least 2 hours or overnight, until the chia pudding has thickened and set.
- Stir the chia pudding before serving to ensure an even consistency.
- Serve the turmeric chia pudding topped with sliced banana, berries, chopped nuts, and shredded coconut for a vibrant and nutrient-packed breakfast option.

4. Vegetable Frittata

Ingredients:

- 6 eggs
- 1/4 cup unsweetened almond milk or dairy-free milk of choice

- 1 cup mixed vegetables (such as spinach, bell peppers, tomatoes, onions, mushrooms)
- 1/4 cup chopped fresh herbs (such as parsley, basil, chives)
- Salt and pepper to taste
- Olive oil or coconut oil for cooking

Instructions:

- Preheat the oven to 350°F (175°C).
- In a bowl, whisk together the eggs, almond milk, salt, and pepper until well combined.
- Heat olive oil or coconut oil in an oven-safe skillet over medium heat. Add the mixed vegetables and sauté until softened, about 5-7 minutes.
- Pour the whisked egg mixture evenly over the sautéed vegetables in the skillet.
- Sprinkle chopped fresh herbs on top of the egg mixture.
- Cook the frittata on the stovetop for 3-4 minutes, until the edges begin to set.
- Transfer the skillet to the preheated oven and bake for 12-15 minutes, until the frittata is set in the center and lightly golden on top.
- Remove the frittata from the oven and let it cool slightly before slicing into wedges.
- Serve the vegetable frittata warm or at room temperature for a protein-rich and veggie-packed breakfast option.

5. Quinoa Breakfast Bowl

Ingredients:

- 1/2 cup cooked quinoa
- 1/2 cup unsweetened almond milk or coconut milk
- 1 tablespoon maple syrup or honey
- 1/2 teaspoon ground cinnamon
- 1/4 teaspoon vanilla extract
- Toppings: sliced banana, berries, chopped nuts, hemp seeds, shredded coconut

Instructions:

- In a small saucepan, combine cooked quinoa, almond milk, maple syrup or honey, ground cinnamon, and vanilla extract.
- Cook over medium heat, stirring occasionally, until heated through and slightly thickened, about 5 minutes.
- Remove from heat and transfer the quinoa mixture to a bowl.
- Top with sliced banana, berries, chopped nuts, hemp seeds, and shredded coconut.
- Serve warm for a hearty and nutritious breakfast option.

6. Sweet Potato Breakfast Hash

Ingredients:

- 1 large sweet potato, peeled and diced
- 1/2 onion, diced
- 1 bell pepper, diced

- 2 cloves garlic, minced
- 1 teaspoon smoked paprika
- 1/2 teaspoon ground cumin
- Salt and pepper to taste
- Olive oil or coconut oil for cooking
- Optional toppings: avocado slices, chopped cilantro, hot sauce

Instructions:

- Heat olive oil or coconut oil in a skillet over medium heat. Add the diced sweet potato and cook until tender and lightly browned, about 8-10 minutes.
- Add the diced onion, bell pepper, and minced garlic to the skillet. Cook until the vegetables are softened, about 5 minutes.
- Season the mixture with smoked paprika, ground cumin, salt, and pepper, stirring to combine.
- Cook for an additional 2-3 minutes, until the spices are fragrant.
- Remove the skillet from heat and transfer the sweet potato hash to serving plates.
- Top with optional toppings such as avocado slices, chopped cilantro, and hot sauce, if desired.
- Serve hot for a flavorful and satisfying breakfast.

7. Coconut Yogurt Parfait

Ingredients:

- 1 cup coconut yogurt
- 1/2 cup granola (choose a variety without added sugar)
- 1/2 cup mixed berries (such as strawberries, blueberries, raspberries)
- 2 tablespoons shredded coconut
- Optional toppings: sliced banana, chopped nuts, honey or maple syrup

Instructions:

- In serving glasses or bowls, layer coconut yogurt, granola, mixed berries, and shredded coconut.
- Repeat the layers until the glasses or bowls are filled.
- Top the parfaits with optional toppings such as sliced banana, chopped nuts, and a drizzle of honey or maple syrup, if desired.
- Serve immediately for a refreshing and nutrient-packed breakfast parfait.

Lunch Recipes
1. Mediterranean Chickpea Salad

Ingredients

- 1 can (15 ounces) chickpeas, drained and rinsed
- 1 cup cherry tomatoes, halved
- 1 cucumber, diced
- 1/4 cup red onion, thinly sliced

- 1/4 cup Kalamata olives, pitted and halved
- 2 tablespoons fresh parsley, chopped
- 2 tablespoons extra-virgin olive oil
- 1 tablespoon lemon juice
- 1 teaspoon dried oregano
- Salt and pepper to taste

Instructions:

- In a large bowl, combine the chickpeas, cherry tomatoes, cucumber, red onion, Kalamata olives, and fresh parsley.
- In a small bowl, whisk together the extra-virgin olive oil, lemon juice, dried oregano, salt, and pepper.
- Pour the dressing over the salad and toss until well combined.
- Serve immediately or refrigerate for later. Enjoy this refreshing and flavorful Mediterranean-inspired salad.

2. Quinoa Stuffed Bell Peppers

Ingredients:

- 4 large bell peppers, any color
- 1 cup cooked quinoa
- 1 can (15 ounces) black beans, drained and rinsed
- 1 cup corn kernels (fresh, frozen, or canned)
- 1 cup cherry tomatoes, diced
- 1/4 cup red onion, finely chopped
- 1/4 cup fresh cilantro, chopped
- 1 teaspoon ground cumin

- 1/2 teaspoon chili powder
- Salt and pepper to taste
- Optional toppings: avocado slices, salsa, Greek yogurt or sour cream

Instructions:

- Preheat the oven to 375°F (190°C). Slice the tops off the bell peppers and remove the seeds and membranes.
- In a large bowl, combine the cooked quinoa, black beans, corn kernels, cherry tomatoes, red onion, fresh cilantro, ground cumin, chili powder, salt, and pepper.
- Spoon the quinoa mixture evenly into the hollowed-out bell peppers.
- Place the stuffed bell peppers in a baking dish and cover with foil.
- Bake in the preheated oven for 25-30 minutes, or until the peppers are tender.
- Remove the foil and bake for an additional 5 minutes to lightly brown the tops.
- Serve the quinoa stuffed bell peppers hot with optional toppings such as avocado slices, salsa, and Greek yogurt or sour cream.

3. Salmon and Avocado Wrap

Ingredients:

- 4 whole grain or gluten-free wraps
- 2 cans (5 ounces each) wild-caught salmon, drained

- 1 avocado, thinly sliced
- 1 cup mixed greens or baby spinach
- 1/4 cup red onion, thinly sliced
- 2 tablespoons Greek yogurt or hummus
- 1 tablespoon Dijon mustard
- Salt and pepper to taste

Instructions:

- Lay out the wraps on a clean surface.
- Spread Greek yogurt or hummus evenly onto each wrap, leaving a border around the edges.
- Divide the drained salmon, avocado slices, mixed greens or baby spinach, and red onion evenly among the wraps.
- Drizzle Dijon mustard over the fillings and season with salt and pepper to taste.
- Roll up the wraps tightly, folding in the sides as you go.
- Cut the wraps in half diagonally and serve immediately or wrap in foil for later. Enjoy this protein-packed and flavorful lunch option.

4. Vegetable and Lentil Soup

Ingredients:

- 1 tablespoon olive oil
- 1 onion, diced
- 2 carrots, diced
- 2 celery stalks, diced
- 2 cloves garlic, minced

- 1 cup dried green or brown lentils, rinsed
- 1 can (14 ounces) diced tomatoes
- 4 cups vegetable broth
- 2 cups water
- 1 teaspoon dried thyme
- 1 teaspoon dried rosemary
- Salt and pepper to taste
- Fresh parsley for garnish

Instructions:

- Heat olive oil in a large pot over medium heat. Add the diced onion, carrots, and celery, and sauté until softened, about 5 minutes.
- Add the minced garlic and cook for an additional minute, until fragrant.
- Stir in the dried lentils, diced tomatoes, vegetable broth, water, dried thyme, dried rosemary, salt, and pepper.
- Bring the soup to a boil, then reduce heat and simmer for 20-25 minutes, or until the lentils are tender.
- Taste and adjust seasoning as needed.
- Ladle the vegetable and lentil soup into bowls, garnish with fresh parsley, and serve hot. Enjoy this hearty and nourishing soup for a comforting lunch.

5. Rainbow Veggie Hummus Wrap

Ingredients:

- 4 whole grain or gluten-free wraps
- 1/2 cup hummus (store-bought or homemade)
- 1 cup mixed vegetables (such as bell peppers, cucumbers, carrots, cherry tomatoes, shredded cabbage)
- 1/4 cup feta cheese or dairy-free cheese (optional)
- Fresh herbs (such as parsley, cilantro, or basil)
- Salt and pepper to taste

Instructions:

- Lay out the wraps on a clean surface.
- Spread hummus evenly onto each wrap, leaving a border around the edges.
- Arrange mixed vegetables and fresh herbs on top of the hummus.
- If using, sprinkle feta cheese or dairy-free cheese over the vegetables.
- Season with salt and pepper to taste.
- Roll up the wraps tightly, folding in the sides as you go.
- Cut the wraps in half diagonally and serve immediately or wrap in foil for later. Enjoy this colorful and veggie-packed lunch option.

Dinner Recipes
1. Grilled Salmon with Lemon Herb Quinoa.

Ingredients:

- 4 salmon fillets
- 1 cup quinoa, rinsed
- 2 cups vegetable broth or water
- Zest and juice of 1 lemon
- 2 tablespoons chopped fresh herbs (such as parsley, dill, or chives)
- Salt and pepper to taste
- Olive oil for grilling

Instructions:

- Preheat the grill to medium-high heat.
- Season the salmon fillets with salt, pepper, and a drizzle of olive oil.
- Grill the salmon fillets for 4-5 minutes per side, or until cooked through and lightly charred.
- Meanwhile, in a saucepan, bring the vegetable broth or water to a boil. Stir in the quinoa, reduce heat to low, cover, and simmer for 15-20 minutes, or until the quinoa is tender and the liquid is absorbed.
- Fluff the cooked quinoa with a fork and stir in the lemon zest, lemon juice, chopped fresh herbs, salt, and pepper.
- Serve the grilled salmon alongside the lemon herb quinoa for a protein-rich and flavorful dinner.

2. Vegetable Stir-Fry with Tofu

Ingredients:

- 1 block extra-firm tofu, pressed and cubed
- 2 tablespoons soy sauce or tamari
- 1 tablespoon rice vinegar
- 1 tablespoon sesame oil
- 2 cloves garlic, minced
- 1 teaspoon grated ginger
- 1 bell pepper, thinly sliced
- 1 cup broccoli florets
- 1 carrot, julienned
- 1 cup snap peas
- 2 green onions, thinly sliced
- Cooked brown rice or quinoa for serving
- Sesame seeds for garnish

Instructions

- In a bowl, whisk together soy sauce or tamari, rice vinegar, sesame oil, minced garlic, and grated ginger.
- Marinate the cubed tofu in the sauce for 15-20 minutes.
- Heat a large skillet or wok over medium-high heat. Add the marinated tofu and cook until browned and crispy, about 5-7 minutes. Remove from the skillet and set aside.
- In the same skillet, add a drizzle of sesame oil and stir-fry the bell pepper, broccoli florets, carrot, and snap peas until tender-crisp, about 5 minutes.
- Return the cooked tofu to the skillet and toss to combine with the vegetables.

- Serve the vegetable stir-fry over cooked brown rice or quinoa, garnished with sliced green onions and sesame seeds.

3. Lentil and Vegetable Curry

Ingredients:

- 1 tablespoon coconut oil or olive oil
- 1 onion, diced
- 2 cloves garlic, minced
- 1 tablespoon grated ginger
- 2 tablespoons curry powder
- 1 teaspoon ground turmeric
- 1 can (14 ounces) diced tomatoes
- 1 can (14 ounces) coconut milk
- 1 cup dried green or brown lentils, rinsed
- 2 cups vegetable broth
- 2 cups mixed vegetables (such as cauliflower, bell peppers, spinach)
- Salt and pepper to taste
- Cooked rice or naan bread for serving

Instructions:

- Heat coconut oil or olive oil in a large pot over medium heat. Add the diced onion and cook until softened, about 5 minutes.
- Add the minced garlic, grated ginger, curry powder, and ground turmeric to the pot. Cook for an additional 2 minutes, until fragrant.

- Stir in the diced tomatoes, coconut milk, dried lentils, and vegetable broth. Bring the mixture to a boil, then reduce heat to low and simmer for 20-25 minutes, or until the lentils are tender.
- Add the mixed vegetables to the pot and simmer for an additional 5-7 minutes, until the vegetables are cooked through.
- Season the lentil and vegetable curry with salt and pepper to taste.
- Serve the curry hot over cooked rice or with naan bread for a comforting and satisfying dinner.

4. Baked Chicken with Roasted Vegetables

Ingredients:

- 4 boneless, skinless chicken breasts
- 2 tablespoons olive oil
- 1 teaspoon dried thyme
- 1 teaspoon dried rosemary
- 1 teaspoon garlic powder
- Salt and pepper to taste
- 4 cups mixed vegetables (such as carrots, potatoes, Brussels sprouts, cauliflower)

Instructions:

- Preheat the oven to 400°F (200°C). Line a baking sheet with parchment paper or lightly grease with olive oil.

- Place the chicken breasts on the prepared baking sheet. Drizzle with olive oil and season with dried thyme, dried rosemary, garlic powder, salt, and pepper.
- Arrange the mixed vegetables around the chicken on the baking sheet. Drizzle with olive oil and season with salt and pepper.
- Bake in the preheated oven for 25-30 minutes, or until the chicken is cooked through and the vegetables are tender and golden brown.
- Remove from the oven and let rest for a few minutes before serving. Enjoy this simple and wholesome dinner option.

5. Eggplant and Chickpea Tagine

Ingredients:

- 1 large eggplant, diced
- 1 can (15 ounces) chickpeas, drained and rinsed
- 1 onion, diced
- 2 cloves garlic, minced
- 1 teaspoon ground cumin
- 1 teaspoon ground coriander
- 1/2 teaspoon ground cinnamon
- 1/4 teaspoon ground turmeric
- 1 can (14 ounces) diced tomatoes
- 1 cup vegetable broth
- 1/4 cup chopped fresh cilantro
- Salt and pepper to taste

- Cooked couscous or quinoa for serving

Instructions:

- Heat olive oil in a large pot or Dutch oven over medium heat. Add the diced eggplant and cook until softened and lightly browned, about 5-7 minutes.
- Add the diced onion and minced garlic to the pot and cook until softened, about 5 minutes.
- Stir in the ground cumin, ground coriander, ground cinnamon, and ground turmeric, and cook for an additional 2 minutes, until fragrant.
- Add the diced tomatoes, chickpeas, and vegetable broth to the pot. Bring the mixture to a boil, then reduce heat to low and

Snack Recipes
1. Hummus with Veggie Sticks

Ingredients:

- 1 can (15 ounces) chickpeas, drained and rinsed
- 2 cloves garlic, minced
- 2 tablespoons tahini
- 2 tablespoons lemon juice
- 2 tablespoons extra-virgin olive oil
- Salt and pepper to taste
- Assorted vegetable sticks (carrots, cucumbers, bell peppers, celery)

Instructions:

- In a food processor, combine the chickpeas, minced garlic, tahini, lemon juice, and olive oil. Blend until smooth and creamy, adding water as needed to reach desired consistency.
- Season the hummus with salt and pepper to taste.
- Serve the hummus with assorted vegetable sticks for dipping. Enjoy this protein-rich and fiber-packed snack option.

2. Greek Yogurt Parfait

Ingredients:

- 1 cup Greek yogurt
- 1/2 cup mixed berries (such as strawberries, blueberries, raspberries)
- 1/4 cup granola (choose a variety without added sugar)
- 1 tablespoon honey or maple syrup (optional)

Instructions:

- In a serving glass or bowl, layer Greek yogurt, mixed berries, and granola.
- Drizzle with honey or maple syrup if desired.
- Repeat the layers until the glass or bowl is filled.
- Serve the Greek yogurt parfait immediately for a protein-rich and nutrient-packed snack.

3. Trail Mix

Ingredients:

- 1 cup mixed nuts (such as almonds, walnuts, cashews)
- 1/2 cup dried fruit (such as raisins, cranberries, apricots)
- 1/4 cup dark chocolate chips or cacao nibs
- 1/4 cup pumpkin seeds or sunflower seeds

Instructions:

- In a large bowl, combine the mixed nuts, dried fruit, dark chocolate chips or cacao nibs, and pumpkin seeds or sunflower seeds.
- Toss to combine.
- Divide the trail mix into individual portions in small bags or containers for easy grab-and-go snacks throughout the week.

4. Stuffed Dates

Ingredients:

- Medjool dates, pitted
- Nut butter (such as almond butter, peanut butter)
- Optional fillings: chopped nuts, dark chocolate chips, shredded coconut

Instructions:

- Carefully slit each date lengthwise and remove the pit.
- Fill each date with a spoonful of nut butter and any optional fillings of your choice.

- Press the edges of the dates together to seal.
- Enjoy stuffed dates as a sweet and satisfying snack.

5. Vegetable Sushi Rolls

Ingredients:

- Nori seaweed sheets
- Cooked sushi rice
- Assorted vegetables (such as cucumber, avocado, carrot, bell pepper, spinach)
- Soy sauce or tamari for dipping

Instructions:

- Place a nori seaweed sheet on a clean surface.
- Spread a thin layer of cooked sushi rice evenly over the nori sheet, leaving a border around the edges.
- Arrange sliced vegetables in the center of the rice.
- Carefully roll up the nori sheet, using a sushi mat or your hands to shape the roll.
- Slice the sushi roll into bite-sized pieces.
- Serve vegetable sushi rolls with soy sauce or tamari for dipping. Enjoy this refreshing and nutritious snack option.

6. Roasted Chickpeas

Ingredients:

- 1 can (15 ounces) chickpeas, drained and rinsed
- 1 tablespoon olive oil

- 1 teaspoon ground cumin
- 1 teaspoon smoked paprika
- 1/2 teaspoon garlic powder
- Salt and pepper to taste

Instructions:

- Preheat the oven to 400°F (200°C). Line a baking sheet with parchment paper.
- Pat the chickpeas dry with a clean towel to remove excess moisture.
- In a bowl, toss the chickpeas with olive oil, ground cumin, smoked paprika, garlic powder, salt, and pepper until evenly coated.
- Spread the chickpeas in a single layer on the prepared baking sheet.
- Bake in the preheated oven for 20-25 minutes, shaking the pan occasionally, until the chickpeas are crispy and golden brown.
- Remove from the oven and let cool before serving. Enjoy roasted chickpeas as a crunchy and flavorful snack.

Green Smoothie

Ingredients:

- 1 cup spinach or kale leaves
- 1/2 banana
- 1/2 cup frozen mixed berries
- 1/2 cup unsweetened almond milk or coconut water

- 1 tablespoon chia seeds or flaxseeds
- Optional add-ins: protein powder, nut butter, Greek yogurt

Instructions:

- In a blender, combine spinach or kale leaves, banana, frozen mixed berries, almond milk or coconut water, and chia seeds or flaxseeds.
- Blend until smooth and creamy.
- Add optional add-ins such as protein powder, nut butter, or Greek yogurt for extra nutrition and flavor.
- Pour the green smoothie into a glass and serve immediately. Enjoy this refreshing and nutrient-packed snack option.

Smoothies and Beverages

Smoothies and beverages are a great way to stay hydrated and nourished while enjoying delicious flavors. Here are seven refreshing and nutritious smoothie and beverage recipes featuring anti-inflammatory ingredients:

1. Tropical Turmeric Smoothie

Ingredients:

- 1 cup frozen pineapple chunks
- 1/2 cup frozen mango chunks
- 1/2 banana
- 1 teaspoon ground turmeric
- 1/2 teaspoon ground ginger

- 1 tablespoon chia seeds or flaxseeds
- 1 cup coconut water or unsweetened almond milk
- Optional: honey or maple syrup for sweetness

Instructions:

- In a blender, combine frozen pineapple chunks, frozen mango chunks, banana, ground turmeric, ground ginger, chia seeds or flaxseeds, and coconut water or almond milk.
- Blend until smooth and creamy.
- Taste and add honey or maple syrup if additional sweetness is desired.
- Pour the tropical turmeric smoothie into a glass and serve immediately. Enjoy this vibrant and refreshing smoothie packed with tropical flavors and anti-inflammatory benefits.

2. Berry Blast Smoothie

Ingredients:

- 1 cup mixed berries (such as strawberries, blueberries, raspberries)
- 1/2 banana
- 1/2 cup spinach or kale leaves
- 1 tablespoon almond butter or peanut butter
- 1 tablespoon hemp seeds or chia seeds
- 1 cup unsweetened almond milk or coconut water
- Optional: honey or maple syrup for sweetness

Instructions:

- In a blender, combine mixed berries, banana, spinach or kale leaves, almond butter or peanut butter, hemp seeds or chia seeds, and almond milk or coconut water.
- Blend until smooth and creamy.
- Taste and add honey or maple syrup if additional sweetness is desired.
- Pour the berry blast smoothie into a glass and serve immediately. Enjoy this antioxidant-rich and nutrient-packed smoothie bursting with berry flavor.

3. Green Goddess Smoothie

Ingredients:

- 1 cup spinach or kale leaves
- 1/2 cucumber, peeled and chopped
- 1/2 avocado, peeled and pitted
- 1/2 banana
- Juice of 1/2 lemon
- 1 tablespoon fresh mint leaves
- 1 cup coconut water or unsweetened almond milk
- Optional: honey or maple syrup for sweetness

Instructions:

- In a blender, combine spinach or kale leaves, chopped cucumber, avocado, banana, lemon juice, fresh mint leaves, and coconut water or almond milk.
- Blend until smooth and creamy.

- Taste and add honey or maple syrup if additional sweetness is desired.
- Pour the green goddess smoothie into a glass and serve immediately. Enjoy this detoxifying and hydrating smoothie filled with green goodness.

4. Golden Milk Latte

Ingredients:

- 1 cup unsweetened almond milk or coconut milk
- 1 teaspoon ground turmeric
- 1/2 teaspoon ground cinnamon
- 1/4 teaspoon ground ginger
- Pinch of black pepper
- Pinch of nutmeg
- Optional: honey or maple syrup for sweetness

Instructions:

- In a small saucepan, heat almond milk or coconut milk over medium heat until warm but not boiling.
- Whisk in ground turmeric, ground cinnamon, ground ginger, black pepper, and nutmeg until well combined.
- Simmer for 3-5 minutes, stirring occasionally.
- Taste and add honey or maple syrup if additional sweetness is desired.
- Pour the golden milk latte into a mug and serve immediately. Enjoy this comforting and soothing

beverage filled with warming spices and anti-inflammatory properties.

5. Beetroot and Berry Smoothie

Ingredients:

- 1 small cooked beetroot, peeled and chopped
- 1/2 cup mixed berries (such as strawberries, raspberries, blackberries)
- 1/2 banana
- 1 tablespoon Greek yogurt or dairy-free yogurt
- 1 tablespoon honey or maple syrup
- 1 cup unsweetened almond milk or coconut water

Instructions:

- In a blender, combine cooked beetroot, mixed berries, banana, Greek yogurt or dairy-free yogurt, honey or maple syrup, and almond milk or coconut water.
- Blend until smooth and creamy.
- Taste and adjust sweetness if necessary.
- Pour the beetroot and berry smoothie into a glass and serve immediately. Enjoy this vibrant and nutrient-packed smoothie bursting with flavor and antioxidants.

6. Chia Seed Lemonade

Ingredients:

- 1 tablespoon chia seeds
- Juice of 1 lemon
- 1 tablespoon honey or maple syrup
- 2 cups water
- Ice cubes
- Lemon slices for garnish

Instructions:

- In a glass or jar, combine chia seeds, lemon juice, honey or maple syrup, and water.
- Stir well to combine and let sit for 10-15 minutes to allow the chia seeds to swell and thicken the mixture.
- Add ice cubes to the chia seed lemonade and stir again.
- Garnish with lemon slices and serve immediately. Enjoy this refreshing and hydrating beverage with a boost of fiber from chia seeds.

7. Pineapple Ginger Cooler

Ingredients:

- 1 cup fresh pineapple chunks
- 1-inch piece of ginger, peeled and grated
- 1 tablespoon honey or maple syrup
- 2 cups water or coconut water
- Ice cubes
- Fresh mint leaves for garnish

Instructions:

- In a blender, combine fresh pineapple chunks, grated ginger, honey or maple syrup, and water or coconut water.
- Blend until smooth.
- Strain the mixture through a fine mesh sieve to remove any pulp or fibers.
- Pour the pineapple ginger cooler into glasses filled with ice cubes.
- Garnish with fresh mint leaves and serve immediately. Enjoy this refreshing and invigorating beverage with a zing of ginger and tropical sweetness.

CHAPTER 6: LIFESTYLE FACTORS

Excellent choice! Lifestyle factors play an important role in reducing inflammation and improving overall health. Here are some significant lifestyle aspects we can look into.

Exercise and Physical Activity:
Regular exercise and physical activity are essential for reducing inflammation and improving overall health. Here's a closer look at the advantages, types of workouts, and strategies for adding physical activity into your daily routine:

The benefits of exercise for inflammation:

- Low levels of inflammatory indicators in the body, including C-reactive protein (CRP) and interleukin-6.
- Increases circulation and blood flow, which can help reduce inflammation in tissues.
- Strengthens the immune system, making it more effective at fighting infections and reducing chronic inflammation.
- Increases the release of endorphins, neurotransmitters that work as natural pain relievers and mood enhancers, thereby reducing stress and inflammation.

Types of Exercises:

- ▷ <u>Aerobic Exercise</u>: Activities including walking, jogging, swimming, cycling, and dancing boost heart rate and promote cardiovascular health. Aim to do at least 150 minutes of moderate-intensity aerobic activity or 75 minutes of vigorous-intensity aerobic exercise each week.
- ▷ <u>Strength Training:</u> Using resistance bands, free weights, or weight machines to improve muscle strength and endurance. Aim for at least two days per week of strength training activities that target key muscle groups.
- ▷ <u>Flexibility and Balance Exercises</u>: Activities like yoga, Pilates, and tai chi increase flexibility, balance, and mobility. Include flexibility exercises in your program at least two to three times per week.

Tips for Integrating Physical Activity:

- ▷ Begin Slowly: If you're new to exercise or have been inactive for a long, start with low-impact activities and gradually increase the intensity and duration over time.
- ▷ Find Activities You Enjoy: Choose activities that you enjoy and are sustainable, such as walking in nature, dancing to music, or participating in sports.
- ▷ Schedule regular workouts. Set out specific times for exercising in your daily or weekly agenda, just like any other important appointment.
- ▷ Mix It Up: Include a variety of exercises in your regimen to keep things interesting and minimize monotony.

Try a variety of workouts, including yoga, hiking, and swimming.

- Listen to Your Body: Notice how your body feels during and after exercise. If you feel pain or discomfort, reduce your intensity or seek advice from a fitness expert.
- Be Consistent: Strive for consistency rather than perfection. Even short bursts of action throughout the day can add up to improve your overall health and well-being.

Note: To incorporate movement throughout the day, take short walking breaks at work or during sedentary activities.

- Whenever possible, use steps rather than elevators.
- Stand up and stretch frequently, especially if you work from a desk.
- Take up an energetic hobby like gardening, dancing, or playing with pets.
- Include physical activity in social gatherings by going on a hike, bike ride, or group fitness class with friends or family.

Stress Management

Chronic stress can promote inflammation and have a negative influence on overall health. Here's an in-depth look at stress management tactics and strategies for lowering stress in your daily life:

1. Mindfulness Meditation:
   - Focus on the present moment without judgment. Regular practice can help to reduce stress, promote self-awareness, and boost general well-being.
   - Begin with short mindfulness meditation sessions and progressively increase the duration as you gain comfort.
   - Start with guided meditation apps or videos, or join mindfulness meditation sessions for further support and instruction.

2. Deep breathing
   - Deep breathing activities, such as diaphragmatic or belly breathing, can promote relaxation and reduce tension.
   - Regularly practice deep breathing exercises, especially during times of stress or tension. - Incorporate deep breathing into your morning routine, before bedtime, or anytime you feel pressured or anxious.

3. Progressive Muscular Relaxation (PMR)
   - Progressive muscle relaxation is the process of tensing and then relaxing distinct muscular groups in the body, which helps to relieve physical stress and promote relaxation.
   - Begin by tensing each muscle group for a few seconds before gradually releasing the tension as you exhale.
   - Work your way from your feet to your head, focusing on how each muscle group feels as you relax it.

4. Yoga and Tai Chi
   - These mind-body practices integrate physical postures, breath work, and meditation to enhance relaxation, and flexibility, and reduce stress.
   - Regularly practice yoga or tai chi to reduce stress, promote awareness, and boost general well-being.
   - Consider taking workshops taught by authorized teachers or watching online tutorials to master proper methods and alignment.

5. Effective time management and prioritization can lessen overwhelm and stress.
   - Break down projects into smaller, more manageable steps and prioritize them according to importance and urgency.
   - Use tools like to-do lists, calendars, and time-blocking techniques to help you arrange your schedule and make time for key activities and self-care.

6. Healthy Lifestyle Habits
   - Regular exercise, a balanced diet, adequate sleep, and avoiding caffeine and alcohol can help reduce the impact of stress on the body.
   - Make self-care a priority by engaging in things that bring you joy and relaxation, such as spending time in nature, pursuing hobbies, or interacting with loved ones.

7. Seeking Support:
   - If feeling overwhelmed by stress, seek help from friends, family, or mental health professionals. - assistance groups, therapy sessions, and stress management programs can all provide useful tools and assistance.

Sleep and Rest.

Quality sleep is critical for general health and well-being, including inflammation control. Here's a closer look at sleep hygiene habits and ways to improve sleep quality:

1. Sleep Schedule
   - Create a consistent sleep schedule by going to bed and waking up at the same times every day, including weekends. Consistency helps to regulate your body's internal clock, resulting in higher sleep quality. The National Sleep Foundation recommends that individuals get 7-9 hours of sleep per night.

2. Establish a Relaxing Bedtime Routine.
   - Set a tranquil routine to communicate to your body that it's time to unwind and prepare for sleep.
   - Relaxing activities include reading, mild stretching, taking a warm bath, and practicing relaxation techniques such as deep breathing or meditation.

3. Optimize Your Sleep Environment:
   - Keep your bedroom cold, dark, and quiet. To minimize distractions, use blackout curtains, earphones, or white noise machines.
   - Invest in a comfy mattress and pillows that provide enough support for your body.

4. Reduce Screen Time Before Bed:
   - Avoid using electronic devices including cellphones, tablets, computers, and TVs in the hour before bedtime. Screens emit blue light, which suppresses the production of melatonin, the hormone that regulates sleep-wake cycles, making it difficult to fall asleep.

5. Maintain a healthy diet and stay hydrated. Avoid heavy meals, coffee, nicotine, and alcohol before bedtime since they might impair sleep.
   - Stay hydrated throughout the day, but limit fluid intake in the hours before bedtime to avoid waking up frequently to use the restroom.

6. Manage Stress and Anxiety:
   - Use stress-reduction strategies like deep breathing, meditation, or progressive muscle relaxation to soothe the mind and body before bedtime.

- Keep a worry notebook to put down any racing thoughts or anxieties before bed, which will help you clear your mind and minimize anxiety.

7. Exercise Regularly
   - Maintain regular physical activity throughout the day, but avoid strenuous exercise near bedtime as it can disrupt sleep.
   - Try to end moderate to severe workouts at least a few hours before bedtime to give your body time to relax.

8. Limit daytime naps to 20-30 minutes. Avoid napping too close to bedtime as it can disrupt evening sleep.

9. Seek practitioner Help if Needed:
   - If you continue to suffer with sleep despite appropriate sleep hygiene routines, talk with a healthcare practitioner or sleep specialist. They can assist diagnose underlying sleep disorders like insomnia, sleep apnea, and restless legs syndrome, as well as prescribe appropriate treatment options.

Supplements and Natural Remedies.
Supplements and natural therapies can help you maintain a healthy lifestyle and manage inflammation. Here's a closer look at some important supplements and natural therapies known for their anti-inflammatory properties:

1. Omega-3 Fatty Acids:
   - Omega-3 fatty acids found in fatty fish (e.g. salmon, mackerel, and sardines), flaxseeds, chia seeds, and walnuts have strong anti-inflammatory properties.
   - Consider taking fish oil or algae oil capsules, which provide concentrated dosages of omega-3 fatty acids, including EPA and DHA.

2. Turmeric and Curcumin:
   - Turmeric, a popular spice in Indian cuisine, includes curcumin, which has anti-inflammatory and antioxidant qualities.
   - Consider taking curcumin supplements or incorporating turmeric into your meals and beverages, such as golden milk or turmeric tea, to gain its anti-inflammatory benefits.

3. Ginger:
   - Ginger has strong anti-inflammatory effects. It includes bioactive chemicals known as gingerols, which have been demonstrated to decrease inflammation and pain.
   - Consider making fresh ginger tea or taking ginger pills to help control inflammation.

4. Probiotics:
   - Probiotics are healthy microorganisms that improve gut health and immunity. A recent study suggests that probiotics may help lower inflammation by fostering a healthy balance of gut bacteria.
   - Consider taking a high-quality probiotic supplement or adding probiotic-rich foods like yogurt, kefir, sauerkraut, and kimchi to your diet.

5. Vitamin D:
   - Vitamin D supports immune function and may reduce inflammation. Many people have insufficient vitamin D levels, especially those who live in northern latitudes or spend little time outside. Consider taking a vitamin D supplement, especially during the winter or if you get little sun exposure, but contact a healthcare practitioner to determine the proper amount.

6. Boswellia (Frankincense):
   - Boswellia serrata, or Indian frankincense, is an herbal supplement derived from the resin of the Boswellia tree. It includes anti-inflammatory chemicals known as boswellic acids. Consider consuming Boswellia pills to help reduce inflammation and relieve symptoms of osteoarthritis and inflammatory bowel disease.

7. Quercetin:
   - Quercetin, a flavonoid found in fruits, vegetables, and herbs, has antioxidant and anti-inflammatory properties.

- Consider eating quercetin-rich foods like apples, onions, berries, kale, and capers, or taking quercetin supplements to help with inflammation management.

8. Green tea:
- Green tea contains polyphenols, specifically epigallocatechin gallate (EGCG), which have powerful antioxidant and anti-inflammatory properties.
- To get the anti-inflammatory benefits of green tea, consider consuming it daily or supplementing with it.

9. Resveratrol:
- Resveratrol, a polyphenol found in red wine, grapes, and some berries, has antioxidant and anti-inflammatory properties.
- Consider eating resveratrol-rich foods or taking resveratrol supplements to help reduce inflammation and improve overall health.

<u>Note</u>:

Before beginning any new supplements or natural treatments, you should check with a healthcare practitioner, especially if you have underlying health concerns, are pregnant or nursing, or are taking drugs, to confirm they are safe and appropriate for your needs. Remember that supplements are intended to augment, not replace, a balanced diet and lifestyle.

CHAPTER 7: PERSONALIZED ANTI-INFLAMMATORY PLAN

A personalized anti-inflammatory approach considers your specific health goals, dietary preferences, lifestyle factors, and any underlying health concerns. Here's how to develop a bespoke plan tailored to your requirements:

Assessing Your Current Diet.

Assessing your current diet is an important first step toward developing an effective anti-inflammatory regimen. Here's how to go deeper into reviewing your eating habits:

1. Keep a food diary
   - Begin by maintaining a detailed food journal for at least one week. Record everything you eat and drink, including portion amounts, meal times, and snacks.
   - Be honest and detailed while noting your dietary intake, including items in homemade meals and beverages.

2. Track symptoms and reactions
   - Take note of any symptoms or reactions you have after consuming specific meals. Bloating, digestive discomfort, exhaustion, joint pain, headaches, skin problems, and mood changes are some of the most common inflammatory symptoms.
   - Look for trends or associations between certain foods or food groups and your symptoms.

3. Assess Macronutrient Balance.
   - Determine the macronutrient balance in your diet (carbohydrates, protein, and fat). Aim for a balanced macronutrient distribution to promote overall health and energy levels.
   - Do you eat enough protein to assist muscle repair and growth? Do you receive enough healthy fats from foods like avocados, nuts, seeds, and olive oil? Are you relying too much on processed carbohydrates or sugary snacks?

4. Evaluate Food Options.
   - Consider the types of things you normally eat. Are you consuming largely whole, minimally processed foods, or do you rely on convenience and fast food?
   - Look for ways to include more nutrient-dense foods like fruits, vegetables, whole grains, lean proteins, and healthy fats in your diet.

5. Identify pro-inflammatory foods.
   - Identify things in your diet that may be pro-inflammatory, such as processed meats, refined carbs, sugary snacks and beverages, fried foods, and foods high in trans and saturated fats.
   - Consider how frequently you eat certain items and how they affect your general health and well-being.

6. Assess Hydration Status.
   - Assess your fluid intake and hydration levels. Do you drink enough water during the day, or do you prefer caffeinated or sugary beverages?
   - Drink lots of water and avoid beverages that can cause dehydration or irritation.

7. Consider Emotional and Environmental Factors.
   - Consider how emotions and the surroundings may influence your nutritional choices. Do you typically eat in response to stress, boredom, or other emotional triggers?
   - Do external circumstances like work schedules, social activities, or travel influence your food preferences and eating habits?

8. Seek Professional Guidance.
   - Consult a trained dietitian or nutritionist, who may evaluate your food diary, assess your eating habits, and make tailored recommendations for improving your diet and reducing inflammation.
   - A healthcare expert can help you discover potential food sensitivities or intolerances, create a personalized nutrition plan, and make long-term dietary modifications.

Goal Setting

Setting goals is essential for success in any effort, including leading an anti-inflammatory lifestyle. Let's look at some ways for setting and meeting your health goals:

1. Reflect on your values and priorities:
   - Begin by reflecting on what is most important to you and what you intend to achieve through your anti-inflammatory lifestyle. Consider your long-term health goals, such as lowering inflammation, increasing energy, managing chronic diseases, or maintaining a healthy weight.

2. Make your goals specific and measurable:
   - Define your goals in clear, explicit language so you know exactly what you're aiming for. Instead of general objectives like "eat healthier," be more precise about what you want to achieve, such as "consume at least five servings of vegetables per day" or "limit processed foods to once per week."
   - Make sure your goals are measurable so you can track your progress and recognize your accomplishments along the way. Set concrete goals, such as "exercise for 30 minutes five days a week" or "reduce sugary beverage consumption to one per week."

3. Break down larger goals into smaller steps:
   - Divide huge tasks into smaller, more doable steps or milestones. This can assist in reducing overwhelm and make progress more tangible and attainable.

- For example, if your objective is to include more physical activity into your routine, begin by setting small goals, such as going for a brief walk after dinner three times a week, then gradually increase the duration and frequency as you gain momentum.

4. Set Attainable and Realistic Goals:
- Set goals that are attainable and practical given your existing lifestyle, interests, and circumstances. Consider time limits, resources, and any roadblocks that may limit your capacity to attain your objectives.
- Be honest with yourself about what you can do in a particular time frame, and don't be hesitant to change your goals as needed.

5. Ensure the goals are relevant and meaningful:
- Make sure your goals are relevant to your specific requirements and consistent with your overall health objectives. Focus on achieving goals that address aspects of your life or habits that contribute to inflammation and overall well-being.
- Select goals that are personally relevant and motivating to you, as you are more likely to remain committed and engaged while working toward goals that align with your beliefs and priorities.

6. Establish Timeframes for Achievement
   - Set clear timetables or deadlines for completing your objectives to instill a sense of urgency and accountability. This could include setting short-term goals (e.g., weekly or monthly targets) as well as long-term goals (e.g., six months or a year).
   - Regularly assess your goals and progress to ensure you're on track and making consistent progress toward your goals.

7. Stay Flexible and Adaptable
   - Be flexible and adaptable in your goal-setting process, acknowledging that priorities and circumstances can change over time. Be willing to revise your goals as needed to keep on track with your changing requirements and desires.
   - Celebrate your accomplishments along the way and avoid being discouraged by setbacks or problems. Use setbacks as chances to learn and grow, and keep focused on your long-term health and well-being goals.

Tracking Progress

Tracking your success is critical to staying motivated and accountable during your anti-inflammatory journey. Here are some techniques to effectively track your progress:

1. Set Clear Metrics
   - Define the measures or indicators you'll use to track your success. This could include changes in symptoms (e.g., decreased joint pain, improved digestion), physical measurements (e.g., weight, waist circumference), dietary habits (e.g., daily fruit and vegetable consumption), or fitness achievements (e.g., enhanced endurance, strength gains).

2. Use a journal or tracker
   - Maintain a dedicated notebook or use a tracking tool to track your daily habits, activities, and progress toward your goals. Record what you consume, how you feel, and any symptoms or improvements you notice.
   - Include information such as portion amounts, meal timings, hydration, exercise habits, and stress levels to acquire an understanding of patterns and trends over time.

3. Track physical measurements
   - Take regular measurements of key physical indicators such as weight, body fat percentage, waist circumference, and blood pressure to track changes in body composition and overall health.
   - Take measurements at regular intervals (such as weekly or monthly) and evaluate your progress over time to uncover patterns and areas for improvement.

4. Keep a food diary.
   - Keep a detailed food journal to monitor your nutritional consumption and find patterns associated with inflammation, digestion, energy levels, and mood.
   - Keep track of everything you eat and drink during the day, including serving quantities, ingredients, and any symptoms or reactions you have.
   - Keep a food diary to identify trigger foods, track your adherence to dietary recommendations, and make changes to your eating habits as necessary.

5. Monitor symptoms and well-being.
   - Monitor changes in symptoms, energy levels, mood, and overall well-being as you follow your anti-inflammatory regimen.
   - Use a symptom tracker or mood journal to note the improvement or worsening of inflammation-related symptoms such as joint pain, digestive troubles, exhaustion, headaches, and skin problems.

6. Celebrate Your Achievements
   - Celebrate your accomplishments, no matter how minor, to stay motivated and encourage great behavior. Recognize your progress toward your goals and be proud of your achievements.
   - Establish prizes for hitting milestones or attaining specified goals to encourage growth and keep momentum.

7. Regularly Review and Reflect
   - Set up regular review sessions to analyze your progress, reflect on your triumphs and problems, and adapt your strategy as appropriate.
   - Use these review sessions to discover areas for progress, establish new goals, and reaffirm your dedication to your anti-inflammatory journey.

8. Seek help and accountability
   - Share your objectives and successes with friends, family, or a support group for motivation, accountability, and feedback.
   - Consult a healthcare practitioner, registered dietitian, or health coach for direction, support, and accountability as you work toward your anti-inflammatory goals.